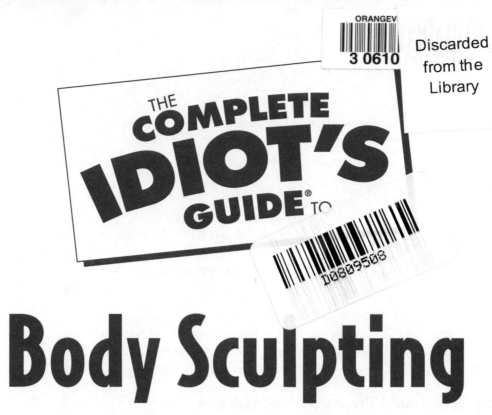

THE COMPLETE IDIOT'S GUIDE® TO

Body Sculpting

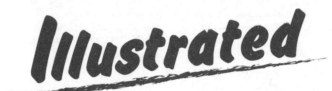

Illustrated

by Patrick S. Hagerman, Ed.D., CSCS*D, NSCA-CPT*D,
with Randall Broderdorf, CPT, and
Jennifer Lata Rung

ALPHA

A member of Penguin Group (USA) Inc.

We dedicate this book to all of you out there who are reading it. You are the ones we wrote this book for. We sincerely hope that you find in it the message you want and the inspiration to achieve the greatness that is in you.

ALPHA BOOKS

Published by the Penguin Group

Penguin Group (USA) Inc., 375 Hudson Street, New York, New York 10014, U.S.A.

Penguin Group (Canada), 10 Alcorn Avenue, Toronto, Ontario, Canada M4V 3B2 (a division of Pearson Penguin Canada Inc.)

Penguin Books Ltd, 80 Strand, London WC2R 0RL, England

Penguin Ireland, 25 St Stephen's Green, Dublin 2, Ireland (a division of Penguin Books Ltd)

Penguin Group (Australia), 250 Camberwell Road, Camberwell, Victoria 3124, Australia (a division of Pearson Australia Group Pty Ltd)

Penguin Books India Pvt Ltd, 11 Community Centre, Panchsheel Park, New Delhi—110 017, India

Penguin Group (NZ), Cnr Airborne and Rosedale Roads, Albany, Auckland, New Zealand (a division of Pearson New Zealand Ltd)

Penguin Books (South Africa) (Pty) Ltd, 24 Sturdee Avenue, Rosebank, Johannesburg 2196, South Africa

Penguin Books Ltd, Registered Offices: 80 Strand, London WC2R 0RL, England

International Standard Book Number: 1-59257-150-6
Library of Congress Catalog Card Number: 2004111428

06 05 04   8 7 6 5 4 3 2 1

Interpretation of the printing code: The rightmost number of the first series of numbers is the year of the book's printing; the rightmost number of the second series of numbers is the number of the book's printing. For example, a printing code of 04-1 shows that the first printing occurred in 2004.

Printed in the United States of America

Note: This publication contains the opinions and ideas of its authors. It is intended to provide helpful and informative material on the subject matter covered. It is sold with the understanding that the authors and publisher are not engaged in rendering professional services in the book. If the reader requires personal assistance or advice, a competent professional should be consulted.

The authors and publisher specifically disclaim any responsibility for any liability, loss, or risk, personal or otherwise, which is incurred as a consequence, directly or indirectly, of the use and application of any of the contents of this book.

Most Alpha books are available at special quantity discounts for bulk purchases for sales promotions, premiums, fund-raising, or educational use. Special books, or book excerpts, can also be created to fit specific needs.

For details, write: Special Markets, Alpha Books, 375 Hudson Street, New York, NY 10014.

Publisher: *Marie Butler-Knight*
Product Manager: *Phil Kitchel*
Senior Managing Editor: *Jennifer Chisholm*
Senior Acquisitions Editor: *Mike Sanders*
Senior Development Editor: *Tom Stevens*
Senior Production Editor: *Billy Fields*
Copy Editor: *Krista Hansing*

Cartoonist: *Jody Schaeffer*
Cover/Book Designer: *Trina Wurst*
Indexer: *Tonya Heard*
Layout: *Becky Harmon*
Graphics: *Tammy Graham*

Contents at a Glance

Contents

Foreword

When it comes to health and fitness, there are no short cuts or easy methods to achievement. As the Director of Education for a nonprofit, international strength and fitness association, I am responsible for maintaining the integrity of the organization on various levels. I am often approached by the latest diet guru or with the latest fitness invention to do what amounts to validating its worth. Infomercials, marketing money, and before-and-after photos all play on the allure of quick-fix results. The truth of the matter is what most individuals need is a clear, nonbias, factual source of information regarding health and fitness.

Dr. Hagerman, Randall Broderdorf, and Jennifer Rung have put together straightforward, factual, and applicable information that everyone who is interested in getting started in a fitness program should read. *The Complete Idiot's Guide to Body Sculpting Illustrated* can be used as a reference guide or training partner. What you won't find is a related diet program you will have to buy forever or a fitness product that will miraculously give you washboard abdominals. What you will find is sensible information that can impact and should be incorporated into most individuals' lives.

The topics selected are the most important for fitness: muscular strength, cardiovascular fitness, flexibility, body composition—and all complemented with nutrition. All the information is broken down and easy to understand. The detail is great, and I especially like the "Extra Rep," "No Pain-Just Gain," "Trainer Talk," and "Q & A."

One of the most impressive sections discusses how the individual should incorporate fitness into one's *lifestyle* by changing habits. Imagine if our country would only do a 30-minute exercise session with a walk or jog instead of munching on junk food and watching television all day. Personally, I would welcome the idea of being known as the world's fittest country instead of the fattest, which we currently are.

The described "Action-Oriented Approach" is tremendous. Write it down, make it a priority, and implement the plan. Realistic objectives are emphasized, which is key for sculpting *your* best physique and benefiting from a fitness program.

My favorite part of this book is the strength-training exercises. If you are truly interested in re-shaping your body, strength training is going to be part of a comprehensive program. Strength training can not only tighten and tone muscles but can also have a positive impact on general health, blood profiles, and health risk factors. The exercises selected and described are excellent for someone getting started. The abdominal training is simple and targeted toward results. If done as described and consistently, the lower body movements are perfect choices and will get the desired effects. Upper body movements don't involve complicated equipment or extensive knowledge to perform. Overall, I have to complement the authors for choosing a menu of outcome-oriented strength-training exercises.

If you are considering starting a fitness program, want to, or already have, you will find this information valuable. I hope that you enjoy this book as much as I do.

—Michael Barnes, MEd, Certified Strength and Conditioning Specialist, NSCA Certified Personal Trainer. National Strength and Conditioning Association, Director of Education

Introduction

Today's fitness and "diet" industry is enormous. Every day you're barraged with ads for the latest gadgets, supplements, and fitness equipment, most of which claim to offer virtually instantaneous results. Most of these claims are based on sketchy information at best; very few are based on sound science.

Body sculpting is different. Body sculpting is proven, time tested, and based on reliable, long-term physiological knowledge. Success is based on four basic components—resistance training, aerobic activity, stretching, and good nutrition. With body sculpting, the sum of the whole is greater than any of its individual parts. It uses information we've understood for many years about all four of these components and puts it together to maximize your body-shaping results.

We don't claim body sculpting will happen overnight. But within a few weeks, you'll begin to notice a significant increase in your strength and energy, not to mention fitter, more sculpted-looking results in the mirror.

This book provides all the tools you need to set up your body-sculpting plan, through resistance training, aerobic activity, stretching, and nutrition. You'll come away from this book knowing how to eat better, how much time you should devote to exercise, and exactly how to incorporate weight training into your exercise plan. The book also explains how it all works, based on proven physiological evidence. By following the advice in this book, you'll be on your way to a fitter, more healthful lifestyle and a body that's the envy of everyone around you.

What You'll Find in This Book

The book is separated into four parts, each of which covers an essential component of your body sculpting plan. **Part 1, "The 'Art' of Body Sculpting,"** explains the basics of body sculpting, including its history and the science that supports it. It also provides you with the tools to develop your own specific body business plan.

Part 2, "Nutrition: The 'Raw' Materials for Sculpting Your Physique," explains the importance of nutrition to body sculpting and provides you with specific information to develop a smart, effective, and satisfying eating plan.

Part 3, "The Building Blocks of Body Sculpting," covers two more essential parts of your body-sculpting program: stretching and aerobic training. In Chapter 7, "Stretching with Ease," you'll find detailed instructions and photographs. In Chapter 8, "Taking Exercise to Heart," you'll learn how to make the most of cardiovascular exercise.

Part 4, "Resistance Training: The 'Tools' for Carving Your Physique," is the heart of the body-sculpting book. In these chapters, you will find all the information you need to maximize your resistance-training program. This information includes step-by-step instructions and photographs of a huge range of resistance exercises to train every muscle in your body.

Throughout the book, you'll also find sidebars with quick and important pieces of information that summarize some of the text or add more information that's important to know. These sidebars include the following:

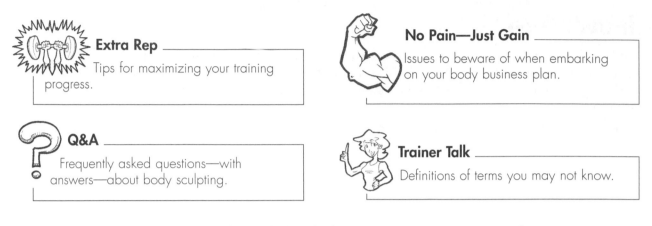

Extra Rep
Tips for maximizing your training progress.

No Pain—Just Gain
Issues to beware of when embarking on your body business plan.

Q&A
Frequently asked questions—with answers—about body sculpting.

Trainer Talk
Definitions of terms you may not know.

So read up, start sweating, and good luck! The key to success is consistency and commitment. We know you can do it!

Acknowledgments

This book was something I had always wanted to do—sort of a long-term goal. Every time a new exercise book came out, I would get it, read it, and gripe about the inaccuracies and problems in it. My wife would always tell me that I needed to write a book that addressed the truth, not the fads. To my wife, Becki, I would like to offer sincere thanks, and of course say "I love you." She pushed me to finally put all my ideas down on paper, put up with the long nights while I worked away, and understood that it was something I had to do my way. She offered encouragement, praise, and a pick-me-up speech whenever it was needed.

To my students and friends who offered to help model for the pictures: This book may or may not lead to a career in front of the camera, but either way, your help was invaluable. A big "thanks" goes to Jay Dawes, Jenifer Anderson, Morgan Francis, Nicole Scott, Mark Sigler, Stephanie Lejbjuk, Aaron Edwards, Jennifer Landrum, and Alicia Pillay.

The University of Tulsa's Collins Fitness Center allowed me to use its facility for the photo shoots and to move its equipment around to make it all work—serious thanks to the staff and management for their cooperation.

Last, but not least, thanks to all those I called upon to be sure the words I wrote made sense. It isn't always easy to get a point across without making it confusing, so I enlisted the help of colleagues and friends to read and reread everything I wrote—and they didn't pull any punches. My co-author, Jennifer Rung, put everything together and offered her professional grammatical advice when I needed it—thanks to you.

Trademarks

In This Part

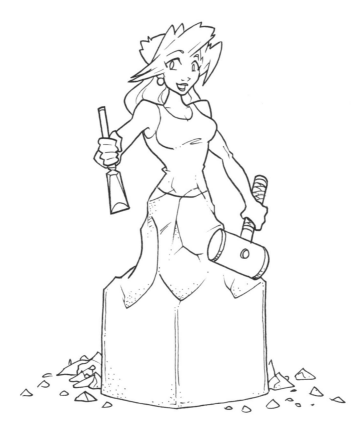

The "Art" of Body Sculpting

If only our bodies were made of clay. It would be so easy to shave a little here, add a little there, and voilà! You'd have the perfect specimen. The bad news is that we can't choose where our excess fat goes. The good news is that, with a little work, we can get rid of it and shape the muscles beneath to become leaner, stronger, and more attractive than before. We do this through body sculpting.

Part 1 explains the history of body sculpting and why it works. It also tells you what to avoid on your quest for a better body, clearing up some of the outlandish myths and bogus product claims you may encounter along the way. Finally, Part 1 gives you the tools and advice you need to develop and stick to an individual body business plan—one that creates the results you desire naturally and healthfully. It's like an extreme makeover, without the extreme methods. What could be better than that?

In This Chapter

◆ Defining body sculpting

◆ Synergy is the key

◆ Genetics and body sculpting

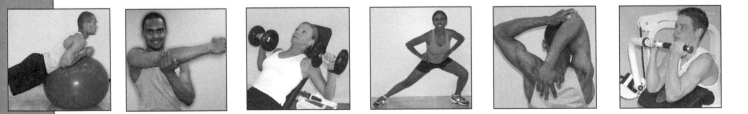

Chapter 1

Just What Is Body Sculpting?

What exactly *is* body sculpting? How does this form of exercise differ from your traditional notions of "shaping up," such as dropping a few pounds, doing aerobics, or running a mile a day?

For many, the phrase *body sculpting* conjures up images of Greek statues or Michelangelo's *David:* flowing lines and perfectly proportioned, well-defined muscles. In reality, the term has a variety of meanings, depending on whom you ask and at what point in time. Simply put, body sculpting means changing the shape of your body in a desirable way. This may include taking a few inches off your thighs, making your shoulder muscles look good, getting rid of those love handles, losing the fat on the back of your arms and replacing it with muscle, or all the above. Just as a sculptor chips away here and adds clay there, think of yourself as the artist and your physique the masterpiece.

Probably the biggest factor that defines body sculpting is its focus on development of lean muscle through resistance exercise. Body sculpting incorporates traditional aerobic exercise as part of a complete program, but resistance training is its cornerstone. By incorporating resistance training into your exercise routine, you will lose weight and inches faster and "sculpt" a toned, fit body that's healthy and strong.

> **Trainer Talk** _____
>
> **Body sculpting** is a philosophy of exercise that incorporates resistance training as part of a complete program to define and tone muscle and shape your body according to your particular goals. For women, this often means losing inches from "problem" areas; for men, it often means gaining inches in areas such as the arms or legs.

Synergy Is the Key

The actual means of achieving a healthy and well-sculpted physique can be summed up in a simple yet powerful concept called *synergy*. Synergy is simply defined as two or more effective components that, when combined, produce an effect that is greater than each of them alone (i.e., 1 + 1 = 3). When you understand synergy and the concepts outlined in this book, you'll be empowered with the knowledge to determine which products and methods of exercise will actually help you achieve the results you're after—and also which ones will lead you to failure. Forget all the fancy, newfangled diets, diet pills, and exercise contraptions; with the power of synergy, four basic components will bring positive, lasting change to your physique:

◆ Proper nutrition

◆ Moderate aerobic exercise

◆ Tension-releasing stretches

◆ Focused, effective resistance training

> **Trainer Talk** _____
>
> The **synergy** of the following four factors is essential to achieving body-sculpting results: proper nutrition; moderate aerobic exercise; tension-releasing stretches; and focused, effective resistance training.

No matter what your condition, goal, experience, or background is, by employing the power of synergy, every single human can achieve a certain degree of results. Essentially, we all burn fat and build muscle in the same way, although to varying degrees, based on a few variables such as genetics. However, if you make modifications to the four components listed—nutrition, aerobic exercise, stretching, and resistance training—you are guaranteed to move toward your goals. This book covers specifics in each of these areas, to help you maximize your results.

The Role of Genetics and Body Type

Someday we may be able to choose which of our genes we'll pass on to our children. But until that time, we'll have to continue shaping our bodies with exercise and nutrition. The role that individual genetics play in our potential for physical development and performance has been the subject of many debates. Although researchers agree that genetics do play a role in how your body can be molded, the question is still, "How much is genetics involved?" Physical traits such as bone and joint structure, muscle fiber count, muscle fiber type, and the location of muscle attachments all play a distinctive role. For the most part, humans all have the same basic structure and physiology, but there are also variations on the basics. It's much like a Cadillac and a Volkswagen Bug: They both have similar parts that allow them to do the same tasks, but, obviously, their looks are quite different.

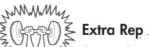

> **Extra Rep** _____
>
> The combination of correct nutrition, flexibility, aerobic exercise, and resistance training will work for everyone, but not everyone's results will be identical. Genetics—and the body you inherit from your parents—also plays a big role.

If you have ever looked closely at professional bodybuilders or models in magazines, you'll notice that even though they may have all achieved an incredible level of development or fitness, they still have noticeable differences. This is due to small differences in their individual structures that come primarily from genetics.

Does Shape Matter?

Research has proven over time that any healthy person can increase muscle mass through overloading the muscles and can support growth and adaptation through sufficient food and nutrient intake. Everybody responds to a body-sculpting style of training, although each person responds differently. We don't all start out with the same body. Some of us have more muscle; some have more fat. It's really all in your genes. This is why the body-sculpting program you use may give your best friend different results.

Is there hope for your body type and genetic background? Absolutely! No matter what cards Mother Nature has dealt you, knowing how to make the most for your unique combination of muscle and metabolism will help you build a sculpture that is bound to turn heads! The rest of this book will help you put that plan together.

The Least You Need to Know

◆ Body sculpting involves the synergy of four essential factors—proper nutrition; moderate aerobic exercise; tension-releasing stretches; and focused, effective resistance training.

◆ Genetics play a distinct role in the ultimate shape of your body; however, by incorporating good habits in nutrition, flexibility, and aerobic and resistance exercise, you *can* maximize your form.

In This Chapter

- ◆ The lure of the quick fix
- ◆ Debunking common exercise myths
- ◆ From low fat to low carb
- ◆ Never too old to act young
- ◆ Mixing up quick-fix potions

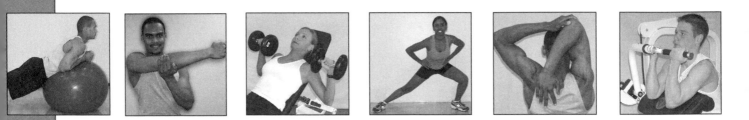

Chapter 2

Separating Fact from Fiction

Extra! Extra! New study shows that exercise is good for you. Next day: Extra! Extra! New study shows that exercise can be bad for you. Everywhere you turn, someone's offering new—and often conflicting—information on diet and exercise. There are countless so-called "experts," and the advice varies as much as the people who offer it. You see it on TV or hear about it from someone in your office or your best friend: Seemingly everyone has a theory on the latest, best way to lose weight and get in shape.

Unfortunately, most of the information floating around the water cooler or being spouted from the TV is wrong. Why would these experts be wrong? Because they were never taught the correct answers, so they just keep telling you what they were told, which was wrong to begin with. It's called *perpetuation of misinformation*. It may sound like the truth, and it may have some confusing explanation that you can't argue with because you don't understand the "science," but it's still wrong. In this chapter, I explain some of the most common misinformation and give you some real ammunition to use the next time somebody tries to sell you a myth. Oh, and by the way, exercise *is* good for you.

Several widely accepted beliefs about exercise and diet are basically untrue. Although the majority of us know deep down that it takes commitment and work to trim and sculpt our bodies, the lure of the "quick fix" just can't be denied. This is especially true when you're presented with emotional testimonials by supposedly real people that this is finally the fix that will take the work out of losing weight or building muscle. Even skeptics of paid infomercials and other advertising have been known to fall victim to various diet and exercise scams—perhaps because we all want so badly to believe there's an easier solution.

Trainer Talk

Perpetuation of misinformation is the term used by true fitness professionals to explain why so many myths are still being accepted as truth. When you understand what is really happening, you can break this cycle.

So what are some of these myths, and what is the truth behind them?

Spot Reduction Fixes Problem Areas

The myth: *Spot reduction* probably tops the list of the most inaccurate body-sculpting promises, yet it still accounts for the majority of exercise gadgets sold today. Spot reducing has become a multimillion-dollar industry in itself. This concept is based on the notion that it is possible to "burn off" fat from a specific region or body part by selectively working that area. Deceptive advertising promises the ability to "take inches off the buns, thighs, waist … all without any effort and only minutes a day!"

Trainer Talk

Spot reduction, or the claim that you can reduce body fat in one specific area of the body by working it with exercises, is a complete myth the weight-loss industry continues to perpetuate. The only way to burn fat is through cardiovascular exercise, and you can't target one portion of the body over another for fat burning.

The truth: Exercising a specific part of the body will *not* stimulate the body to use fat from just that area. Think of fat like blood. If you cut your finger, you don't get finger blood; you

get blood. The fat on your midsection isn't midsection fat; it's body fat. Resistance exercise stimulates increases in muscular strength, endurance, or size in the muscles you train. Doing sit-ups or squeezing your thighs together will not eliminate fat from those areas, but it will make those muscles stronger and more sculpted. For years, people have purchased these "state-of-the-art" gadgets or gravitated toward certain exercise machines in the gym in an effort to "tone" their flabby areas. But body flab—a.k.a. fat—can't be sculpted. The muscle *underneath* the flab can be sculpted, so spot exercising isn't completely useless. The only way you'll see the results of this muscle sculpting, however, is to first burn off the fat that is covering up the muscles. And the only way to eliminate body fat is by doing cardiovascular exercise and making sure you eat fewer calories than you burn.

Nature's cruel little trick (actually, thousands of years of evolution) is that most people store excess calories as body fat concentrated in certain spots of the body. In men, this tends to be in the trunk area of the abdomen and chest. In women, it tends to be predominately in the lower extremities of the hips, glutes, and thighs.

But this is where nature doesn't play fair. Although we tend to store body fat predominately in certain areas, how much fat is burned from each area is genetically predetermined. Unfortunately for those of us who want to target a specific area, fat is usually lost evenly throughout the whole body. So even if you've got a higher amount of fat on your stomach than anywhere else, your body will burn the same percentage of fat from your stomach as it does from your arms, legs, back, and rear end. So as you are losing fat in your stomach, you are also losing fat on your arms, calves, and hips. The result is that our "problem areas," or those areas with more fat, are often the last to see all the fat go away. But don't despair: If you are consistent and don't give up, you will eventually see all the excess fat disappear from your problem areas. When your body has removed all the excess fat from those areas you are not targeting, then it has no choice but to take it from wherever there is fat left.

Lifting Weights Will Make Me Bulky

The myth: Many women have stayed away from resistance training because they don't want to end up looking like a man or like the female bodybuilders they see on TV. It's easy to see why the myth may have started—before fitness centers became common, they were called gyms, and these were predominantly the lair of weight-lifting men. Because we didn't have enough science to understand that men and women react differently to resistance training, it was assumed that a woman would get bigger muscles and become more "manly" if she lifted weights. This myth has continued today partly because of the growth of female bodybuilding.

The truth: The mere act of engaging in resistance training will not make you big and bulky. Actually, the amount of muscle mass you can build depends on the type of training you do (sets, reps, and load), the amount and type of calories you take in (and burn), your sex, and your genetic makeup, among other things. Any time you lift weights and do resistance training, your muscles are becoming stronger—but not necessarily bigger.

The reason men tend to gain muscle size is simply because they have more testosterone. Testosterone is an anabolic (building) hormone that everyone produces, but men have about 10 times more testosterone in their bodies, so they are able to build more muscle. For this reason, women shouldn't fear training with weights. Besides, if it were so effortless to build huge slabs of muscle mass merely by lifting weights, you would see many more massively built men walking around everywhere! Even for the average guy with all those anabolic hormones, it is still a challenge to build large, hulking muscles.

Aside from the hormones, the amount of training and effort required for a female to get muscles the size of a professional bodybuilder is much more than most of us are willing to expend. Professional female bodybuilders usually lift weights for several hours a day, have a very strict diet, and usually do not have a healthy amount of body fat. Even if you wanted to get into professional bodybuilding, your genetics will have some say in it. Only a small percentage of the population can reach the most elite ranks of muscle development, and they require the right combination of resistance training, hormones, and genetics.

For the average person trying to "lean out" and sculpt their physique, there is no more effective or faster way of changing body shape than doing resistance training. So put aside any fears you may have about getting too big by starting a body-sculpting program. The program details in this book are designed not to build big muscles, but to give flattering definition to the muscles you have.

 Extra Rep

Because fat cells take up more room than muscle cells in the body, replacing fat with muscle will make you appear only leaner, not bulkier, as the myth holds.

Turning Fat into Muscle (and Vice Versa)

The myth: Many people believe that toning and building muscle involves turning fat cells into muscle cells; if you stop exercising, therefore, muscle will turn back into fat. This is a prominent myth that has no basis.

The truth: Muscle and fat are two completely different tissues, and one cannot become the other. It's like saying that you can paint an apple orange, and it becomes an orange. It's still an apple—with orange paint. This particular belief continues, often due to the perception of athletes who suddenly stop working out. When well-muscled athletes or bodybuilders decrease the intensity and amount of strenuous exercise in their lives—or they stop exercising altogether—they often continue to eat the same amount of calories they ate during their exercising days. They are eating more than they are burning off (because they are not exercising as much anymore), so the extra calories get stored as fat. Additionally, by reducing their exercise, they inevitably lose muscle mass and definition, giving them that flat, "sagging" look. Adjusting their caloric intake to match their activity level—and making exercise an integral part of their lifestyle—combats this scenario.

In the same light, if you carry excess body fat, you can change the composition of your body by engaging in resistance exercise. Fat is burned in the muscles, so building lean mass helps burn off the layers of fat. Remember, muscle burns calories and fat, but fat just sits there. If you increase the amount of active muscle, you burn more calories and fat. If you increase the amount of fat, you just get more fat. In most cases, you don't have to increase the size of your muscles to burn more fat; you just have to make the muscles you have more active. We all have muscle that is not working at its full potential for fat burning. With body-sculpting exercises, you make your muscles stronger and more efficient at burning fat, without promoting a lot of bulk.

When you get the sculpted physique you want, you can maintain your body shape with less exercise than it took to get it, without having to worry about losing the muscle and gaining back fat. Numerous studies show that light to moderate strength training for each muscle group just one time a week helps you maintain

the gains you made and keep your "engine" burning fuel at optimal levels. We'll talk more about this later.

Extra Rep

When you increase the amount of lean muscle in your body, you increase the amount of calories you burn, even when your body is at rest. This is why resistance training is an integral part of weight loss.

Workouts Have to Be Hard and Frequent

The myth: Some fitness fanatics claim that if you don't work out hard for at least an hour every day (and don't even think about taking a day off), you won't make any progress, so you might as well not even start. This sort of thinking is ridiculous! Many people believe that a workout has to be hard and frequent to exhibit any results. This mind-set would keep most rational people from even starting an exercise program.

The truth: Any exercise is better than no exercise at all. I like to tell people who bring up this misconception, "A little bit of something is better than a whole lot of nothing!" If you are reading the bodybuilding magazines and notice that their workouts last two to three hours, or two hours twice a day, remember that these people are working toward something totally different than you are. Research shows that any kind of activity, such as brisk walking, gardening, or a quick 10- to 15-minute body-sculpting weight circuit as infrequently as once a week will reduce the risk of diseases.

For our goals, body sculpting does require at least a commitment of three times a week, but even if you occasionally miss a day, you can always make it up. Body sculpting will never be an all-or-nothing issue. The beauty of body sculpting is that you can actually have a job and a life outside your workouts and still get results!

I'm Too Old, So It's Too Late

The myth: Some people believe that only twenty-somethings can improve their physiques. They think, "I'm no spring chicken, so I'll never be able to get into better shape."

The truth: It is never too late to experience the many benefits of exercise. In fact, many of the problems associated with aging are due to a lack of activity—not necessarily aging in and of itself. True, hormone levels reduce as we age, recuperation time may be lengthened, and various precautions should be taken. However, we can still experience increases in muscle mass, strength, and function, as well as reversal of many ailments associated with aging.

As an example, one of my clients, age 88, had never exercised before she came to see me. She came in only because her daughter brought her. At first she could not get off the couch or out of a chair without help. Her legs had gotten weak because of inactivity. It took only six weeks of regular exercise to get her muscles back in shape so she could get up by herself. After 5 years of exercise, she was doing squats, lunges, and step-ups without any problem—at age 93. The moral of the story is this: By exercising, you can actually add a few years to your life span—and you'll improve your quality of life during those years. Plus, you'll have a sculpted look that will make others envious!

Specially Engineered Foods and Protein Formulas Build Muscle Faster

The myth: The premise behind specially engineered foods and formulas is that they can miraculously help you build muscle mass at a faster rate. You'll find these types of marketing statements in droves on the pages of bodybuilding and exercise magazines. Beautifully sculpted bodies on the labels portray the idea that, by drinking this drink, eating this energy bar, or swallowing these pills, you'll reach your goal more quickly.

The truth: No dietary protein or special formula will initiate faster muscle building (also known as hypertrophy). Only appropriate exercise supported by proper nutrition will help build muscle. If you eat a balanced diet, there is no nutritional advantage to consuming special whey protein formulas over other complete proteins, drinking special (and often terrible-tasting) drinks during the day, or eating "scientifically designed" bars rather than real food. Muscle is built at its genetically predetermined pace, as long as proper overall nutrition is combined with appropriate exercise.

The Least You Need to Know

◆ There's no such thing as spot reduction for a specific region of the body.
◆ Lifting weights to reach your specific goals will not make you bulky.
◆ You don't have to give up everything else in your life to achieve and maintain a lean, well-muscled physique.
◆ You're never too old to begin an exercise program.
◆ There are no magic potions or secret formulas for losing fat or gaining muscle.

In This Chapter

- ◆ The newest infomercial gizmo
- ◆ Abdominal machines and electrical muscle stimulators
- ◆ Pills that burn and block fat
- ◆ How fad diets can hurt, not help

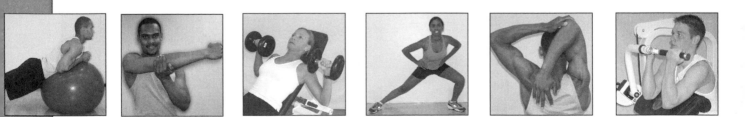

Chapter 3

Buyer Beware!

There's the co-worker who lost 10 dress sizes with new a breakthrough diet that involves eating only 2 types of food that miraculously burn fat. Then there's the gal on the afternoon talk show who claims she can eat anything—in any quantity—and still lose weight just by taking a "fat-blocking" pill. And we mustn't forget the relative who lost weight by eating according to his blood type—and only at odd hours, but never when the moon is full. Sounds ridiculous, doesn't it? Even so, you may have tried one or more of these methods or diets yourself. That's okay. If you have tried any "too good to be true" methods, you already know that they don't work for very long. In our quest to achieve a slim and trim physique, we sometimes lose touch with common sense and become victims of our own desperation. This is exactly what most of the purveyors of these dubious diets and gizmos prey upon—and make huge amounts of money from!

Unfortunately, a very large majority of those who try these fad pills and diets find their search for the "weight-loss holy grail" continuing on and on and on. Most of these diets, supplements, and exercise gizmos have sketchy scientific data to support their claims—if there's any data at all. But it's often easy to believe them. After all, aren't we protected by "truth in advertising" laws? And wouldn't we have heard already if that supplement really was just snake oil?

This chapter sheds some light on the most popular gizmos and gimmicks out there. Of course, there is no way to cover each and every gimmick available, especially when new ones are introduced almost daily. Most fall under one basic category, so by arming yourself with correct scientific information and a little common sense, you'll be able to spot the snake oil salesman miles away.

No Pain—Just Gain

Don't believe everything you see on TV or in magazines. Product claims are often made with no proven data to support them. In fact, the Food and Drug Administration (FDA) has recently been taking legal action against weight-loss products that promise more than they deliver.

Exercise Gizmos and Magic Bullets

We've all seen them: late-night "infomercials" that peddle the latest, greatest, until-now-a-secret, rapid-weight-loss gadgets and supplements that are guaranteed to give you a firm, tone, sculpted, fat-free, and younger body in just three minutes a day. We're also inundated with product marketing as we flip through magazines, such as "before and after" photos of "everyday" people who have achieved unbelievable results using product X. Or we see bodybuilders professing that the latest "breakthrough" supplement was the element largely responsible for creating their physique, even if the product was just recently manufactured and introduced.

Most of us have become conditioned to be mildly entertained—and, for the most part, skeptical—of this marketing and advertising. But there's also a small part of us that wonders each time we see one of these ads, "What if *this* is finally the thing that gets me into shape?"

Enough people in the United States listening to that little voice have turned the weight-loss industry into a nearly $40 billion-a-year business. Yet according to a study in the *Journal of the American Medical Association*, the obesity rate in the United States is currently estimated at almost one third (31 percent) of the entire U.S. population as of 2002, up from 23 percent in 1994 and 15 percent in 1980. Nearly 64 percent of Americans are either overweight or obese.

How can this be, when the weight-loss industry is constantly providing us with the latest and greatest products that promise quick and easy results? Projections estimate the industry to grow by 5.6 percent annually—right along with America's waistline.

Abdominal Trainers

Abdominal trainers claim to be able to spot reduce—that is, eliminate fat specifically from your stomach and midsection. The truth is, doing hundreds or even thousands of sit-ups will not cause you to lose fat from your midsection (remember, we talked about this in Chapter 2). This is especially laughable when you consider that most of these devices claim that they can help in just minutes a day, without any effort and absolutely no sweating! By using such a device, you might build stronger abdominal muscles, but they will still be covered with body fat. Except for the novelty of having a nifty contraption to use while working the abdominal region, there is no advantage to using one of these gizmos over doing simple sit-ups or crunches.

Extra Rep

The only way to see defined muscles is to burn off the fat that covers them. This means that no matter how strong your abdominal muscles are, you'll never see that six-pack if you're carrying excess abdominal fat.

Weight-Reducing Clothing

Special weight-reducing exercise garments, such as sweat belts and rubberized suits, are still big sellers, although not as popular as in years past. These garments do two things: They make you sweat, and they squeeze your fat into a smaller area. You do lose weight when you sweat, but you are not sweating fat. When you sweat, you lose mainly water, which is universally considered to be fat free. This means that you have reduced your weight but not your fat, leaving you with a higher percentage of body fat than before because you lost "lean" weight instead of fat weight. This dehydration is caused by fabrics that trap heat and decrease the airflow that cools your body. Also, because these garments are usually very tight, the localized pressure causes tissue compression (stuffing the fat into a smaller area). Although weight may be temporarily reduced using these garments (until rehydration occurs) and circumference measurements may be briefly condensed due to compressing fat tissue below the skin, these results are short lived and unrelated to actual or lasting reductions in body weight or fat stores.

I once had a client who, before working with me, wore a rubberized suit while exercising. He actually ran and lifted weights with the suit on and then did sit-ups in the dry sauna, thinking that this would help burn more body fat. The exercise probably did help him lose body fat, but the rubber suit just made him sweat more, causing him to lose water weight as well. He could always see immediate results on the scale after his workout because it's very easy to drop two to three pounds of water weight. Unfortunately, after he went home and had a few glasses of water, his weight was back to where he started. The next day, he started all over again. It took some convincing and patience, but he eventually let go of the emotional attachment to this potentially dangerous practice. He ended up dropping the body fat he had been trying to lose through more effective body-sculpting methods.

Electrical Muscle Stimulators

The promotion of electrical muscle stimulators (EMS) has become popular over the last couple years. Advertisements claim that by strapping one of these devices onto a flabby body part,

"microelectroimpulses" provide the same sculpting effects as doing 3,000 sit-ups or jogging 10 miles—with no effort at all! The science behind these devices is convincing because all muscles are activated through electrical impulses. Although EMS devices are used in certain therapy applications for chronic disease and related medical conditions, numerous studies conducted over the years have shown no benefits to using such devices for bodybuilding and muscle definition. In fact, the FDA has recently taken action against companies that make outlandish and unrealistic claims about EMS products, labeling them fraudulent.

In addition to the deceptive claims, EMS devices can be potentially hazardous if misused. Potential complications can include burns and electric shocks. If a strong current passes through the brain, heart, or spinal column, life-threatening consequences are even possible.

Fat Blockers

Wouldn't it be convenient to be able to take a pill and eat whatever you wanted, knowing that you wouldn't absorb any dietary fat into your system? Promoters of fat-blocking supplements tout special ingredients such as carnitine, St. John's wort, synephrine, chromium, and a marine fiber called chitosan. These ingredients supposedly bind to ingested fat, making the molecule too large to be absorbed through the small intestine and, thus, eliminated by the body. Without exception, research has failed to confirm the effectiveness of these substances.

Some brands of snack products have even included a "fake fat," known by the shelf name Olestra (or Olean). Problems associated with eating foods containing Olestra include abdominal cramping and distress; anal leakage; loose stools; and problems absorbing vitamins A, D, K, and particularly E. Originally, Proctor and Gamble had hoped this product would take the place of all cooking oils and dietary fat, but

Olestra was relegated for use only in snack products after problems with the FDA. Sales of products containing Olestra have declined steadily since the late 1990s.

Fat Burners

One of the most widely selling supplements in recent years has been an herbal fat burner, sold under various brand names such as Metaboost and Zantrex3. The primary ingredient is a naturally occurring form of ephedra (or ephedrine) called mahuang. Ephedra is a potent stimulant that is also the base compound for methamphetamine (a.k.a. speed), which affects the nervous and cardiovascular systems. The mahuang is usually blended with caffeine or its herbal equivalent, guarana, and other stimulants that can cause symptoms such as increases in heart rate and blood pressure. Although evidence may suggest that these stimulants promote modest weight loss in some individuals, this substance has been linked with a number of deaths and other serious documented reactions, such as chest pain, seizures, and heart attacks.

To date, no long-term studies have indicated how dangerous these products could prove to be. However, with all the negative press about the use of such supplements, many products that did have ephedra in them modified their formulas to exclude it—and this pretty much makes them useless. Some retailers refused to sell ephedra-containing products to minors or pulled these brands from their stores completely. A number of sports organizations, including the National Football League, National Collegiate Athletics Association, and International Olympic Committee, have banned the use of products containing ephedra. Finally, because of potentially life-threatening side effects when taking ephedra-containing products, in April 2004, the FDA banned any and all ephedra products in the United States.

No Pain—Just Gain

The American Heart Association has warned that ephedra's possible side effects far exceed any weight-loss benefits. Complications such as high blood pressure, irregular heartbeat, seizures, heart attack, and stroke have been associated with ephedra use.

Steroids

Anabolic-androgenic steroids are man-made substances related to the male sex hormone testosterone. These drugs are available legally only by prescription and are used medically to treat conditions that occur when the body produces abnormally low amounts of testosterone, such as delayed puberty and some types of impotence. They are also used to treat the loss of lean muscle mass in patients with AIDS and other diseases.

Trainer Talk

Anabolic-androgenic steroids were developed for medical purposes, to normalize the amount of testosterone in the body. *Anabolic* refers to muscle building, and *androgenic* refers to increased masculine characteristics. *Steroids* refers to the class of drugs. Over the years, their abuse has grown by athletes and bodybuilders seeking to enhance the natural effects of training. Unfortunately, the use of steroids can cause severe, even life-threatening side effects.

Today, athletes and others abuse anabolic steroids in an effort to enhance performance and improve physical appearance. Unfortunately, this abuse can lead to serious health problems, some irreversible. Anabolic steroids are taken orally or injected, typically in cycles of weeks or months rather than continuously. Major side effects of abusing anabolic steroids include liver tumors and cancer, jaundice (yellowish pigmentation of skin, tissues, and body fluids), fluid retention, high blood pressure, increases in LDL (bad cholesterol), and decreases in HDL (good cholesterol). Other side effects include kidney tumors, severe acne, and trembling. There are also some unpleasant gender-specific side effects:

◆ **For men.** Shrinking of the testicles, reduced sperm count, infertility, baldness, and increased risk for prostate cancer.

◆ **For women.** Growth of facial hair, male-pattern baldness, changes in or cessation of the menstrual cycle, and deepened voice.

◆ **For adolescents.** Growth can be halted due to premature skeletal maturation and accelerated puberty changes. If teens take anabolic steroids before the typical adolescent growth spurt, they can risk remaining short the rest of their lives.

In addition, if needles are shared, people who inject anabolic steroids run the risk of contracting or transmitting HIV/AIDS or hepatitis. Scientific research also shows that aggression and other psychiatric side effects may result from abuse of anabolic steroids. Many users report feeling good about themselves while on anabolic steroids, but researchers report that extreme mood swings, including maniclike symptoms leading to violence, can occur. Depression often results when the person stops taking steroids, which may contribute to chemical dependence on anabolic steroids. Researchers also report that users may suffer from paranoid jealousy, extreme irritability, delusions, and impaired judgment stemming from feelings of invincibility.

Anabolic steroids do work, but at what cost? Needless to say, the health and legal risks far outweigh any benefits associated with steroid use.

Cellulite Creams

Cellulite is simply a fancy name for fat. A significant portion of the body's fat is stored subcutaneously (directly beneath the skin), where strands of connective fiber separate fat cells into compartments. When the fat cells expand, they protrude out of these compartments, giving the skin a dimpled appearance. Unfortunately, nothing as simple or as superficial as a cream could possibly break down or reverse the process of fibrosis. There has yet to be any scientific evidence that herbal lotions or strange potions wear down anything but a hole in your pocketbook. These creams and lotions seem to work because they can cause the skin to *temporarily* become more hydrated, or actually bloated, thus hiding the dimples.

They're Called *Fad* Diets for a Reason

Wouldn't it be great if we could follow some new "breakthrough" diet plan and quickly and easily have a lean, well-chiseled physique that would turn peoples' heads in admiration? As with most things, if it sounds too good to be true … you know the rest. Quick-fix gimmicks simply do not address the causes of weight gain or lack of muscular definition, so they are temporary fixes, at best. Most of the time, they are completely ineffective and possibly even dangerous to your health. Think of it this way: If any one of these techniques actually worked, everyone would be using it and everyone would look great. Unfortunately, this is not the case. As I stated before, the population is becoming more out of shape and overweight than ever.

The key to achieving muscular definition, reaching a healthy body weight, and maintaining both is to adopt a lifestyle that is conducive to such goals. Look around at the people you see who have the type of body you want to have. They are probably eating right and exercising properly, not using one strange gimmick after another. Going on and off fad diets, battling with excess weight, then resorting to drastic measures to quickly and temporarily lose it is not only unhealthy, it's no way to live your life. The key is to effectively implement lasting changes that make it possible to keep your sculpted form for the long haul.

All in all, subjecting your body and psyche to continued abuse with gimmicky, "quick-fix" diets is no way to obtain and keep a sculpted body. Sometimes it takes several attempts before you are ultimately successful in achieving and maintaining a lean physique—the healthy way. And that's all right. Learning what is effective and what is merely marketing gimmickry is the first step in developing a plan that's effective for you. To make it easier, ask yourself this question before you start a new program: "Is this something that will fit into my lifestyle, not make me feel deprived, and something that I will be able to do for the rest of my life?" If the answer is no, then don't start it.

Inaccurate beliefs, myths, and fads flourish because the public as a whole has very little accurate information about proper fat loss and muscle gain. This allows sensational, faddish methods to gain popularity. Old miracle diets are revived, and new miracle diets are invented constantly. While people continue to look for a magic bullet, marketers search for new gimmicks to prey on the public's desperation and increase their profits. Let's look at some of the more popular fad diets and weight-loss and muscle-gaining gimmicks that are rampant today.

Low-Carbohydrate Diets

The Zone, Sugar Busters, Dr. Atkins' New Diet Revolution, The Carbohydrate Addict's Diet, The South Beach Diet, and Protein Power are just some of the latest fad diets that tell you that the fastest way to lose weight comes from reducing or eliminating carbohydrates from your diet. To begin with, there is a lot of controversy surrounding the validity and long-term health risks of eating a diet extremely low in carbohydrates.

Here's the theory: Carbohydrates cause spikes in blood-sugar (glucose) levels and have the propensity for being easily stored as body fat if they are not burned. As glucose levels rise, the pancreas releases insulin to send sugar to the brain and into the muscles, and the excess gets stored as fat. The thinking is, if you eat more protein and fat and limit your intake of carbohydrates, you'll avoid the rapid rise in blood sugar, so there is less sugar to be stored as fat. These diets also claim that, by eating a high-protein/high-fat diet, the body will metabolize fat in lieu of carbohydrates to provide energy. However, there is no scientific evidence to support such claims and theories.

Let's take a closer look at what actually takes place with this type of eating pattern. Besides being the body's preferred source of energy, carbohydrates are stored in cells as glycogen. Glycogen storage requires lots of water, which hydrates much of the body and increases the cells' efficiency (hence the name carbo*hydrate*). By consuming large quantities of protein and fat and limiting carbohydrates, the cells don't store much glycogen. Without glycogen, there is no need for water, so that water is moved out of the cells, making them dehydrated and less efficient. All this water loss causes your body weight to go down. The problem is that the weight loss is, again, water, not fat. So although you are losing weight, your percentage of body fat has actually increased!

Also, by limiting such a large number of foods because they contain carbohydrates, you are essentially simply on a lower-calorie diet. Think about it. If 50, 60, or 70 percent of your calories are coming from carbohydrates and you suddenly remove them from your diet, you almost certainly will experience weight loss. I know what you're thinking: "It sounds great for getting ready for that reunion or vacation coming up!" But we're after real, long-lasting, healthful results—not yo-yo dieting.

No Pain—Just Gain

Because the health risks of certain diets are not yet fully known, it's best to avoid them. The most effective way to lose weight and build muscle is to eat a diet that correctly balances proteins, carbs, and fats. See Chapters 5 and 6 for specific guidelines.

The potential health risks associated with this type of eating regimen are numerous. Almost anyone who has ever tried one of these diets can tell you how lethargic and irritable he or she became. This occurs because the brain is deprived of its favorite food: blood sugar from carbohydrates. In addition, there is evidence that kidney problems may develop due to the presence of increased ketone bodies, which are produced as a result of poor glucose metabolism. These ketone bodies are usually caused by starvation or diabetes. Furthermore, if too few carbohydrates are available for energy, the body breaks down proteins—either from the diet or muscle tissue—to supply the energy it needs. This extra process is not only inefficient, but it takes away from your muscles' ability to replenish and get ready for your next workout.

Blood sugar must also be present to efficiently fan the flame that burns body fat. Hitting the "wall," a term often used by endurance athletes to describe the depletion of glycogen stores, renders them unable to continue intense physical activity even though body fat is present. Think of it this way: Fat provides energy, so if we could just burn fat, then we should be able to exercise continuously until we have burned off all our excess fat. It doesn't work that way, does it? We get tired after exercising a while because we have run out of glycogen, or carbohydrates, even though we have fat left. When you are out of carbohydrates, you're done. You can't exercise efficiently and burn fat anymore without using your body's protein. So if you are on a low-carbohydrate diet, you won't be able to exercise as long and, thus, will not burn as many fat calories.

You get the idea. Besides, who can sanely maintain such a restrictive diet? We discuss the role of proper nutrition in detail in Chapters 5 and 6.

Blood Type Diet

The Blood Type Diet maintains that eating incorrectly for your specific blood type results in certain diseases and that the body heals itself and burns off body fat when it is fed the fuel it was designed to utilize via evolution. The problem is that your blood doesn't know one food from another. The food you eat doesn't go to your blood; it goes to your stomach to be digested. Nutrients from the digestion process are absorbed into the blood and delivered to where they need to go. The blood is merely the bus that delivers the calories to the muscles, or to the fat cells for storage, if there are too many. That's it; that's its job. Your blood doesn't discriminate between different types of food; it is an equal-opportunity transporter.

One-Food Diets and Other Crazy Ideas

For many people, these diets tend to be a last-ditch effort when a special event is coming up and time is running out. The Cabbage Soup

Diet, the Grapefruit Diet, the 3-Day Diet, the 7-Day All You Can Eat Diet (of one food type, that is), the Caveman Diet, the Hollywood Diet, the One Good Meal Diet—I could go on and on. These extremely restrictive and low-calorie diets promote rapid weight loss simply because you are *temporarily* eating less than you are burning off. Claims that cabbage soup is a "fat-burning soup" or that following a one-food diet will "cleanse" the body should not be believed. Unfortunately, eating cabbage soup, grapefruits, or any one food combined with a few select others doesn't promote well-being because you will not be able to get all the various vitamins and nutrients your body needs for healthy functioning. A friend of mine who works in Hollywood as a personal trainer to a lot of big-name actors and actresses tells me that there is no such thing as a "Hollywood diet" that makes all the celebrities look good. It all comes from simple body-sculpting principles and proper nutrition.

These crackpot diets wreak havoc on your body, metabolism, and health, and can actually cause your body to become increasingly resilient to fat loss. You may lose a few pounds quickly, but chances are good that you'll gain back those pounds—and more—when you've finished the diet. Following the suggestions throughout this book will pleasantly make these diets bad jokes of the past.

If the Yo-Yo Goes Down, It Comes Back Up

Have you tried the "yo-yo" diet? The yo-yo effect is the repeated process of weight loss followed by weight gain, also known as weight cycling. Weight cycling is most common in those who significantly restrict calories to lose weight and then gain back the weight when their calorie intake returns to normal. It has been reported in the popular press, as well as in professional literature, that yo-yo dieting

can lead to several negative physiological, medical, and psychological consequences.

These consequences can include a reduction in lean body mass, an increase in body fat percentage, a chronic lowering of the resting metabolic rate (the number of calories your body burns at rest), an impaired glucose tolerance, and increased blood pressure. This method of dieting also reportedly causes negative effects on mood and self-esteem. It has even been thought to alter what's known as a person's *set point*. Your set point is the weight your body is comfortable maintaining and fights to stay at. Your set point is mainly determined by your genetics (again, something you cannot change), but yo-yo dieting seems to increase your set point. Each time you lose weight and gain it back again, you gain a little bit more than you started with. This is your body's way of protecting itself from losing too much weight. It's thinking, "I'm about to start another diet and lose too much weight too fast. I'd better store up some extra fat to keep from getting too low." Additionally, by continually losing and gaining weight, some experts believe that your body becomes more resistant to losing weight each successive time you diet.

Trainer Talk

Your body's **set point** is the weight that your body is comfortable maintaining. Yo-yo dieting has been associated with increasing the body's set point, making it more difficult to reach weight-loss goals.

The Secrets of "Magic" Revealed

As you can see, even with all the nifty gadgets available, there is still no magic substitute for sensible eating, regular exercise, and a little common sense. Any good magician will tell you that what looks like a simple trick actually took a lot of consistent work and learning to get it right. The reason Americans are getting heavier has not been due to a *lack* of contraptions and newfangled diet plans, but rather *because* of them. They distract people from adopting methods that will help them lose weight and build muscle in a realistic fashion.

Simply put, Americans are increasing in width due to an increase in the number of calories they consume and a decrease in their activity levels and movement. Ironically, all the great advancements in technology that have improved the quality of our lives have also fostered weight gain and structural and postural problems. So pay attention the next time you see a new product advertised that promises to "melt away the pounds" or "tone, trim, and firm." Listen carefully to the next person you encounter touting the latest great diet invention. Then try placing it into one of the categories I've mentioned in this chapter. Chances are, it'll fit into at least one, and that voice of sanity and reason will tell that little desperate voice to get real (or get your money back).

The Least You Need to Know

◆ Infomercial exercise gizmos are not the end-all, be-all of fitness. They usually lighten your wallet more than your body.

◆ Only exercise can burn calories. Cellulite creams, fat-burning pills, electrical stimulators, and rubber suits either hide the problem or make it worse.

◆ Low-carbohydrate diets prevent you from being able to exercise efficiently and only cause you to lose water weight.

◆ Any diet that restricts you to a few select foods deprives your body of complete and proper nutrition.

◆ Stick to the old adage: If it sounds too good to be true, then it probably is.

In This Chapter

- The S.M.A.R.T. way to setting sculpting goals
- Setting long-term and short-term goals
- Changing your habits to match your goals
- Visualizing your goals to stay focused

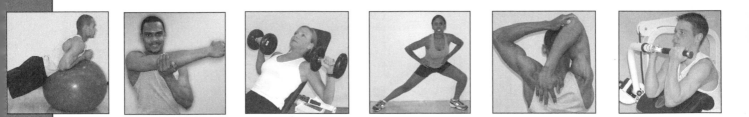

Chapter 4

Developing Your Body Business Plan

In the first three chapters, we discussed the definitions of a sculpted body, as well as the role of genetics and body type. We also looked at many of the quick-fix gimmicks and unsuccessful means of diet and exercise available today. Now that you understand some of the basics, it's time to start outlining the steps necessary to achieve fat loss and muscular definition in your quest for a well-defined body.

In reality, acquiring and maintaining a lean shape really isn't all that complicated. The real challenge is balancing exercise and healthful eating habits with your current lifestyle, which often includes the following:

- ◆ Working stressful jobs with mounting demands and hours
- ◆ The increasing expectation and desire to achieve a standard of living that requires, in most cases, at least two incomes to sustain
- ◆ Kids with as many obligations and responsibilities as their already-overburdened parents
- ◆ Lack of physical activity in everyday life, due to the multitude of machinery designed to save time and effort
- ◆ A higher percentage of sedentary occupations
- ◆ Leisure activities that don't include exercise
- ◆ Easy access to fast food and overly processed convenience foods

Add them up, and you have America's current recipe for something that looks more like a glob of clay than a lean, sculpted physique. To change this and give yourself the body you really want, you have to do some planning and organizing before you start making changes in your eating and exercise. As the saying goes, "He who fails to plan, plans on failing."

Success Is Spelled S.M.A.R.T.

Overcoming these lifestyle realities involves creating a clear plan with an ongoing, effective set of steps to get you there. This is where we develop what I like to call your body business plan. Think of your fitness goals as if you were going into business. You start with a vision: a sculpted, lean, muscular, and well-toned body. This is your long-term goal—it's where you see your business ending up. But how do you get there? And when you get there, how do you hold on to everything you've worked so hard to achieve and continue to build upon it? To reach your long-term goal, you first set up some short-term goals. As another old saying goes, "Every journey begins with the first step."

First, consider the following questions: What do you hope to accomplish with your workouts and eating habits in the next six months? How about the next year? And the following three years? Is this the year you are finally going to lose 20 pounds? Do you want to fit back into your size 6 clothing? What about building those lean, 16-inch arms you've been dreaming about? Or what about that ever-elusive six-pack for the summer? These are all great long-term, basic goals, but to get you there, you'll need to break them down into plans with smaller, specific targets.

You begin by setting short- and long-term goals. We'll do this the S.M.A.R.T. way. Each step in the S.M.A.R.T. process is designed to help you form your overall body business plan

that will guide you in defining and achieving your goals. These steps include the following:

- ◆ Specific goals
- ◆ Measurable methods
- ◆ An action-oriented approach
- ◆ Realistic objectives
- ◆ Time-stamped results

Specific Goals: Deciding What You Want

You probably wouldn't start chipping here and chiseling there on a block of granite without an idea of what you wanted to create. The same holds true for your physique. To achieve a goal, you first must conceive that goal. Instead of merely thinking "I want to have a sculpted body" and then doing some exercises in hopes that somehow it just happens, you'll want to create specific objectives. You need to have a long-term goal (your finished masterpiece) and several smaller short-term goals that basically break down your long-term goal into tiny pieces.

Extra Rep

To achieve a goal, you must first conceive that goal. When setting out to create a leaner physique, you should set specific long- and short-term goals.

It is also important to determine what lies behind your specific goals. For instance, let's say your long-term goal is to lose 10 pounds. *Why* is that is your goal? Has someone else told you that this is what you should lose? Are you trying to weigh what you did in college? Or does some chart tell you that as a 5-foot, 2-inch female, you need to weigh 115 pounds or be considered overweight?

Consider this: What if you were to gain 5 pounds of muscle and lose 10 pounds of fat, thereby significantly reducing your body fat percentage but not seeing much change in your scale weight? If you had more energy and more stamina, felt and looked better in your clothes, and could wear that strapless number for your upcoming reunion, wouldn't this be more motivating than just "losing 10 pounds"? By examining the underlying reasons for your desire to change your body, we're attempting to uncover your *driving want.*

Trainer Talk

> Your **driving want** is the underlying emotional motivation for achieving your body-sculpting goals. You may find, after discovering your driving want, that your goal actually changes. For instance, instead of "losing 10 pounds," it may be "replacing body fat with muscle mass."

This emotional underpinning is the strongest motivation in achieving your goal. Perhaps what you want is not really a lower number on the scale, but what goes along with achieving it: the energy and sense of well-being that come from exercise and eating healthfully. Or maybe it's the admiration of your friends and the opposite sex that truly motivates you. By examining your driving want, you might find that your true goal is now completely different than your original: Your weight is just fine, but you really want to tone your muscles, reduce body fat, and increase muscle mass. It is just as important to know why you want to achieve something as it is to know what you want to accomplish.

Your long-term goal may be a subjective feeling or an objective look you're going for, but your short-term goals should be concrete steps that will take you along this new path.

Specific short-term goals look like this:

◆ I will reduce my intake of dietary fat by 135 calories per day within 2 weeks.

◆ I will commit to resistance exercise at least 30 minutes 3 days per week for the next 3 months.

◆ I will include aerobic work on my lunch break three days per week.

Measurable Methods: Charting Your Progress

By knowing specifically what you want, you will be able to measure whether you are indeed on the road to achieving it. Defining and envisioning your idea of a sculpted physique—before you begin working to achieve it—is essential to achieving your end goal. But you'll also need to measure your progress and know how to determine when you have arrived. The mirror can be a good source of feedback, but in the beginning stages of your program, it may not give you the whole story. Changes to your appearance may take a little while to notice (especially when you see yourself every day), so the mirror may not be the best tool to indicate that changes are actually taking place. Instead, you should develop methods to measure your progress that include not just your changing weight on the scale but also determining body composition, taking circumference measurements, keeping an exercise and eating log, doing strength/endurance charting, and more. The point of setting measurable goals is to ensure that you can tell on a weekly or monthly basis whether you are making progress or whether you need to adjust your exercise and eating routines.

If your goal is simply to be "healthier," it will be more difficult to assess when you have actually reached your goal. Your concept of good health probably differs greatly from everyone else's. However, you will be able to recognize general improvements in your energy level, overall wellness, and even mental health through exercise. And although you can't necessarily measure them with scientific tools such as a scale or a tape measure, you'll be able to determine your success through anecdotal evidence such as better sleep, less fatigue, and fewer illnesses.

These are some examples of measures you can use to evaluate your progress:

◆ I have reduced the number of snacks I eat every day from three to one.

◆ I have exercised at least three times each week for the past month.

◆ I have lost two inches from my waist and one inch from my hips over the last six weeks.

◆ I have increased the amount of weight I can use on my bicep curls and leg press by 25 percent.

◆ I have increased the time I can jog without getting out of breath by 10 minutes.

◆ I have lost one pound of fat each week.

An Action-Oriented Approach: Steps to Get You There

Knowing what you want and making sure you're getting there is effective only if you're following through with the activities necessary to see results. For instance, a goal of reaching 10 percent body fat by losing a pound of fat a week and gaining 2 pounds of muscle a month is specific and measurable, but now you have to determine the steps you need to get there. This is where you construct your action plan. What sort of cardiovascular workout will you need to do? How often? What changes do you need to make in your eating habits? What strength-training program will help build muscle or reduce body fat? This book is designed to help you construct an action plan with the specific activities that will help you achieve your goals. We go into the

details of how to put together your exercise program in Chapters 8 and 9.

Realistic Objectives: *David* Wasn't Carved in a Day

"I don't want to wait years for my chiseled physique. Just tell me what exercises to do and what to eat *now!*"

One of the most overlooked—and most important—steps in this process is to adopt a realistic attitude so you don't get discouraged or give up. Certainly, keeping your goals within the realm of possibility is one of the most difficult things to do, especially when you're constantly bombarded with product ads that claim they'll help you lose weight and look perfect in days or weeks. Losing 15–20 pounds in a month is not only unrealistic, but it also could be dangerous.

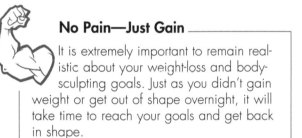

No Pain—Just Gain

It is extremely important to remain realistic about your weight-loss and body-sculpting goals. Just as you didn't gain weight or get out of shape overnight, it will take time to reach your goals and get back in shape.

A plan that consists of 20 minutes of aerobic exercise plus 20 minutes of resistance exercise 2–3 times a week is an example of a realistic starting point. On the other hand, if you're a beginner who sets a goal of four to six days of aerobic exercise and four days of strength training per week, you may be less likely to achieve your goal. You should design your plan around the rest of your life. Your exercise and nutritional strategies should be able to coexist with all the other activities you are involved in every day. For instance, if your plan includes cooking all your meals and not eating out, but you have only enough time to cook once a day, you will need to either figure out how to fit that goal into your life or change your activities to fit the goal. It's great to have big dreams, but all dreams start with small steps. Dream big, but plan carefully.

Having realistic and achievable goals will greatly increase your chances for success and decrease the risk that you will become frustrated and give up altogether. This doesn't mean that you cannot experience great results in a short amount of time, but in today's society, we tend to want everything yesterday. Being realistic about your results as well as your goals is critical for making sure you stick with a progressively sound plan for ultimate results! I can promise you that you will get the body you want, but you have to be consistent and patient and understand that changes aren't always visible in the mirror. Many positive body-sculpting changes are taking place inside your body. Think of it as a process that works from the inside out.

Time-Stamped Results: Setting Dates for Your Achievements

Adhering to a specific time frame always brings the most effective results: graduating college in four years, paying off a mortgage in 20 years, losing two inches from your midsection in four months. Without this last step—time-stamped results—your goals are simply daydreams, "someday" wishes.

Attaching a deadline to each of your goals will help motivate you when your inspiration begins to wane. Write them down. Put them on your calendar, and remind yourself daily of your commitment, your goals, your actions, and your progress. Tell friends and family who are supportive of your goals so they can encourage you. When you know other people

are expecting you to accomplish goals, it can provide additional motivation to stick to your plan.

Staying S.M.A.R.T.

To reach your long-term goal, you should review your short-term goals on a regular basis. Try setting daily behavior goals, such as drinking more water, skipping those beers after work, or making sure you get to sleep at a decent hour.

Next, set some weekly goals, such as exercising 3 times, cutting out or adding 150 calories each day (which adds up to 1,050 for the week), or adding additional time to your aerobic workout. Try setting goals for the first three months and then establish new goals for the next three months. These short-term goals and accomplishments will set the stage for your long-term goal of a sculpted body.

But before you even begin setting your goals and modifying your behaviors, you'll need to track your current eating and exercise behaviors to determine what needs improving. Recognizing these patterns and behaviors, and developing alternatives, is the first step in effectively turning them around.

Extra Rep

If at first you don't succeed, try again. An ongoing examination of your goals and behaviors is necessary to determine whether you're actually achieving what you've set out to do. If you haven't seen progress, it may be time to modify your short-term exercise and eating behaviors.

Life Is Habit Forming

The chances for success in achieving your sculpted physique depend not only on proper and consistent goal setting, but also on your behaviors and approach to food and exercise. One of the great challenges in changing your lifestyle is to change your unhealthful eating and exercise habits, or behaviors, into healthful, consistent habits.

You need to know exactly what needs fixing before you decide to fix it. It may seem apparent that "I need to lose weight," but what you need to discover is what has caused you to need to lose weight. Have you been eating too often or too much? Not exercising consistently? Not exercising the right way? Or is it something else? Examine your lifestyle up to this point. How did you arrive here? What decisions have contributed to the shape your body is in now? How can you change them? These are the questions that will help you put it all in perspective, get on the right track, and stay there.

Has This Habit Gone Bad?

The first step to adopting more positive habits is to identify what you're doing now by keeping a food and exercise log. Write it down! Simply keep track of the type and amount of food you eat every day and the type and amount of exercise you engage in. By keeping a food and exercise log, you won't forget about the soda or bag of chips you ate, or those few Hershey's Kisses you popped into your mouth after passing by the receptionist's desk. And you'll feel accountable when you write "watch TV" instead of "30 minutes on the StairMaster" that you had planned on doing. A log will also identify your habits by telling you when and how much you ate, which is just as important as defining *what* you ate. Plus, logs don't lie. Instead, they increase awareness about what you're eating and how you're exercising.

> **No Pain—Just Gain**
>
> To keep a food and exercise log properly, be sure to document everything in detail: what you ate, how much you ate, and what time you ate it. Also write down the amount and type of physical activity per day (be sure to include nontraditional exercise, such as gardening and vacuuming). And don't forget to log those on-the-go treats and snacks!

Tracking your food consumption and logging your exercise will help you identify your lifestyle patterns, which will help you understand why and when you eat and exercise. This, in turn, will help you correlate eating and exercise patterns with mood, activities, places, and even people—like your buddy, who loves to order double rounds of beer and french fries whenever you guys hang out. A sample food and exercise log is shown in Appendix D.

Probably many triggers in your life drive you to either snack or overeat, and the greatest sculpting exercises in the world will do little to help you achieve your goals if you don't change these habits. For example, if your nightly reality-TV fix always seems to involve chips or ice cream, you're probably eating out of habit rather than hunger. To reach your goals, you will want to break the habit or replace your goodies with a more healthful snack.

When it comes to exercise, tracking exactly what you do in your workouts—and when you actually do or don't exercise—will help uncover influences or lack of motivation that may need to be addressed. The biggest excuse I see for not doing the exercise that was planned for that day is "I got so busy that I ran out of time." We all have the same number of hours in a day to work with. How we decide to use those hours is what makes one person successful and keeps another person struggling to get it together.

Keep a log of not only what exercise you do, but when you do it, how you felt about it (whether you felt rushed or used it as a time to relax and concentrate), and, if other things seemed more important than exercise, what those were. This will help you understand how your daily life is affected by exercise, and how exercise affects your daily life. If you consistently find yourself writing down that you didn't find time to exercise, then you should examine what is taking all your time. My favorite retort to people who say they don't have enough time to exercise is "If the president of the United States can jog five times a week, you can find time in your schedule, too."

It has been proven that those who consistently monitor food consumption and exercise lose weight and gain muscle more steadily—and maintain results more successfully—than those who don't monitor their behavior. Even fitness professionals keep activity and food logs because there is always room for reflection and improvement.

Be a Habit Handyman

Which takes more work, breaking a bad habit or starting a good habit? Actually, they both take the same amount of time. Research has shown that the first seven days of change are the hardest, but that if you stick to it for three weeks, it becomes a habit. In the grand scheme of things, three weeks is very little time. You can do anything for three weeks—and if you can do it for three weeks, you can do it for the rest of your life (hint: that's how you maintain your new sculpted body when you get it).

Identifying your habits and deciding which ones are bad is the first step to changing; however, this alone will not alter your behavior. Developing alternatives to combat bad habits when they occur is the second step. You should have a game plan that will give you direction each time a bad habit tries to rear its ugly face. For instance, one of the most common bad habits I've seen is eating when you are not hungry. To combat this habit, have some alternative activities ready to keep you busy until the urge passes:

◆ Work in the garden.

◆ Pop in an exercise tape and work up a sweat.

◆ Read a good book or magazine (an exercise book can be inspiring!).

◆ Go for a walk or jog.

◆ Take a bubble bath.

◆ Do push-ups or jumping jacks, or skip rope.

◆ Play cards or a board game.

◆ Get together with a friend or spouse to talk, not eat.

◆ Do housework or laundry.

◆ Wash the car.

◆ Bathe the dog or cat.

◆ Write an e-mail or letter to a friend.

◆ Do any other pleasurable activity or necessary action until the urge passes.

You get the picture. The point is to find something constructive and conducive to creating the lifestyle that helps achieve and maintain the body you want.

If you can't seem to totally eliminate a bad habit, you can at least make adjustments to improve it. For instance, if one of your bad habits occurs during that midafternoon energy slump at the office—and there's not much you can do besides sit at your desk and keep working—make the necessary adjustments to modify your habit. Instead of going to get candy, cookies, or chips from the vending machine to carry you through, plan ahead and bring some more healthful snacks. These should be snacks you enjoy: If plain celery sticks won't satisfy you, bring some low-fat Wheat Thins with reduced-fat cheese.

When you are able to better understand what your bad habits are, you can make more healthful choices in the future—and see better results. However, you'll never know if you've made the "right" choices if you can't review them, so write down everything in your food log—and keep it up, even after you begin changing your habits.

If You Can See It, You Can Achieve It

One of the most vital components for achieving success in any endeavor is to effectively set goals. Even if you know all the best exercises, the proper foods to eat, and the top-notch supplements to take, without proper goal setting—and holding yourself accountable for reaching this goal—you will probably never achieve the physique you have in mind. I can't stress this enough: If you don't know where you're going, you will never get there.

We all have goals, whether we realize them or not. Making a conscious effort to recognize them so we have control over their outcome is important to achieving them—and also to keep them from controlling us. You can start using effective yet simple methods *today* to help you set new goals and actually achieve them. Then you will finally obtain the sculpted body and better quality of life you have envisioned for so long.

No Pain—Just Gain

It's natural to experience a setback while pursuing your goal. The key is to learn from your mistakes and modify your behavior to overcome obstacles in the future.

The Journal of a Lifetime

The first step, which I want you to start today, is to spend just 10 to 15 minutes each day writing down your goals in a journal or notebook. Start out asking yourself, "What do I want to achieve? What would I do and how would I feel if I knew I could not fail?" Think of this as your wish list for Christmas; nothing is too outlandish, and nothing is too much to ask for! Feel the excitement start to grow. For our purposes, let's say your goal is to achieve a sculpted physique. Your next step is to write down seven things you can do this week to begin achieving that goal. Be very specific—remember, that's the first step in S.M.A.R.T. goal setting. State exactly how much fat you want to lose or how much muscle you want to add, and specify the steps you need to take to get there.

Next, take a couple minutes and write a paragraph stating why you are now absolutely committed to achieving this goal (and you thought the only work you had to do was lift weights!). Remember, this is your moment to shine, to achieve something extraordinary. Take action!

Reflect on Success

Each evening, when things have wound down and you have some quiet time, open your journal and review what you have written on previous days. Reread your goals, your "why" paragraph, and the action steps you've outlined. Picture them vividly in your mind. Close your eyes and visualize them, as if they were in a movie you just watched. Imagine yourself completing an intense exercise routine, and feel how invigorated you become. Envision yourself eating the tastiest, most healthful foods; how good they make you feel; and how much more energy they provide you with. Picture yourself with power and control, turning down all the fatty junk foods that will do nothing for your new and exciting vision of yourself. Think of how eating donuts, french fries, and desserts are something "ordinary" people do—not the owners of sleek, chiseled bodies. If being ordinary led to such a look, everyone would possess what seems to be so elusive. Feel the sense of confidence, control, pride, and excitement you'll have knowing you are actually doing it. Imagine how you will feel, how people will see you, and how you will inspire others around you as a leader and someone who has taken charge of his or her life.

When you have done the visualization for about five minutes, write down three things you did that day that brought you closer to achieving your goals. Then write down two things you could have done better. Make a commitment to improve on these weak-link areas in the coming days and weeks.

Keep It in Focus

To stay focused and continue visualizing your goals, post pictures of things that remind and inspire you. Put them somewhere you will see them often. This might be a photo of yourself at your "ideal" weight, a photo of someone you admire, or pictures of healthful snacks. Place them on your fridge, in your office, on your nightstand, or in your briefcase or purse. Visualize yourself with a new body as you do the things you do everyday: working, walking, or seeing someone you haven't seen in a while. Get excited!

Expect and plan for setbacks and challenges—they will come. How you deal with them determines your ultimate success. "Failures" often provide you with valuable insight into how you need to adapt. Being flexible gives you the power to find new, possibly even better approaches.

Extra Rep

Goal setting and visualization are absolutely critical to success. They are tools top professionals and leaders in many fields have credited for their achievements.

Have fun, set your goals, get excited, and get ready to make the most incredible progress in the next few weeks and months you ever have made in your life! This is your time, and the time is now. You are capable of achieving tremendous things!

The Least You Need to Know

◆ Our lifestyles and habits are often not conducive to losing weight and gaining muscle; we must change our habits to achieve success.

◆ The S.M.A.R.T. approach to body sculpting involves creating a clear plan with an ongoing, effective set of steps to achieve your goals.

◆ To achieve a long-term goal, you should develop short-term goals to follow on a daily basis. This could mean cutting a certain number of calories, eating better foods, or adding cardiovascular or resistance exercise.

◆ The only way to achieve a goal is to set a concrete objective, track your progress, and visualize your success.

In This Part

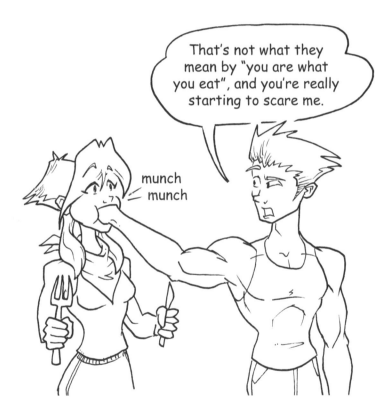

Nutrition: The "Raw" Materials for Sculpting Your Physique

One day we hear that grains are good for us; the next they're considered evil incarnate. When it comes to nutrition, it's tough to know what to believe. The next two chapters dispel the myths surrounding nutrition with sound scientific knowledge to arm you with the information you need to make healthful and nutritious dietary choices. These choices are also aimed at maximizing your body-sculpting program, providing the energy you need to work out and the building blocks you need to strengthen muscle and burn fat. It's simple information with huge potential to give you the results you're seeking: strength, good health, and a more sculpted physique.

In This Chapter

◆ What are calories, and why does your body need them?

◆ The right balance of carbohydrates, proteins, and fats

◆ How vitamins, minerals, and supplements fit into your body business plan

◆ The importance of staying hydrated

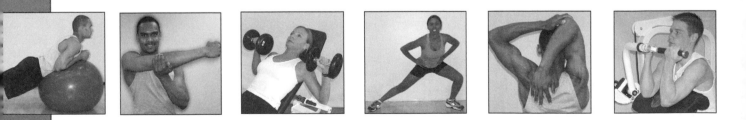

Chapter 5

Feeding the Body

Everywhere you turn nowadays, someone is dishing out nutritional advice. Eat this, don't eat that, be sure you get enough of this. What you put in your body has a lot to do with what you get out of your body—so in many ways, the old saying "You are what you eat" is really true. We want sculpted bodies, so we have to feed ourselves in a way that promotes muscle building and fat loss. We need to focus on the foods we can use to build muscle and burn for energy instead of store as fat. This doesn't mean we can't eat fat; as I've said before, fat is an important part of our diets. What we do need to look at, however, is exactly what we are eating over a period of time. To maximize our dietary intake, we must first understand what we are eating and then figure out how these things affect our bodies.

Dietary advice is so common that there is absolutely no way everyone can be right. There are countless experts and so-called "experts," and just as many conflicting ideas about what's healthful and what isn't. A true nutritional expert is a registered dietician, also called an R.D., who has a degree in nutrition and has passed a professional examination.

No Pain—Just Gain

Like exercise, nutrition is based not on mystery, but rather on pure science. The key to good nutrition, and a diet that helps you reach your body-sculpting and health goals, is based first on knowledge and second on follow-through.

That said, I confess that I am neither a nutrition expert nor a registered dietician. But you don't have to be an expert to understand the basic science that governs how the body uses food to create energy and how excess energy is stored as fat. This chapter and the next cover just the basics of nutrition—the irrefutable science that is the basis of all current thinking in nutrition. These basics are always the same, no matter who is talking, so beware of those peddling diets who claim to have a "secret" never before revealed. The information I'm going to arm you with is basic knowledge that any registered dietician will back up. It's information you can use to define the dietary side of your body business plan.

What's a Calorie?

It seems that everyone is worried about calories. Advertisements for new foods often claim they have fewer calories than other foods. I like calories. In fact, you can't live without calories. A calorie is just a measure of energy that has been adopted as a simple way for us to compare foods. For instance, if a cupcake has 100 calories and an apple has 100 calories, then they provide the same nutritional value, right?

Most of us are armed with enough information to know that an apple and a cupcake are not created equal. Sure, they both have 100 calories, but the cupcake has more calories from fat than the apple (which is mainly carbohydrate calories). So even though they both have 100 calories, those calories are not all the same. And even though the 100 calories in that cupcake may taste much better than those in the apple, this example shows us that basing our diets simply on a food's number of calories doesn't help much in deciding what foods to eat.

You can find calories in three places: carbohydrates, fats, and proteins. Collectively, they are called nutrients because their calories provide energy. If a food doesn't fall into one of these categories, it doesn't have any calories. So if some newfangled diet food is supposed to be calorie free, it's safe to say that it doesn't have any carbohydrates, fats, or proteins (which makes you wonder what you're actually ingesting). Things such as water, vitamins, herbs, spices, chemicals, and prescription drugs don't contain any calories because they aren't made of carbohydrates, fats, or proteins.

Remember that a calorie is a unit of energy, so zero calories means zero energy. Any calorie-free food or drink is also energy free. I'm sure you've seen products that are supposed to give you lots of energy or boost your energy. But without any carbs, fats, or proteins, they can't do that—there is no source of energy. These products are usually full of chemicals and "natural" ingredients that may help the body in other ways we don't know about yet, but they don't provide energy.

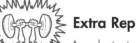

Extra Rep _____

A calorie is simply a unit of energy. No calories = no energy. That's why calories are absolutely necessary to provide the energy you need to maximize your cardiovascular exercise and resistance training.

Now for the complicated part: The three nutrients don't all provide the same number of calories per gram of food. A gram of carbohydrate or protein has 4 calories, and a gram of fat has 9 calories. With some simple math, we can deduce that a gram of fat has more than twice the number of calories as a gram of carbs or protein. If you put 100 calories of fat on a plate and 100 calories of carbohydrates or protein on a plate, the fat portion would be very small, and the carb/protein portion would be much larger. For example, 1 tablespoon of butter (which is 100 percent fat) is 100 calories, and 1 cup of grapes is 100 calories (100 percent carbs). Fat takes up less room. Don't think a food can't have many calories in it because it's really small (such as a candy bar).

Fill 'Er Up with High Octane

To sculpt your body, you need the right fuel. Think of your body as a high-performance race car. If you put cheap fuel in a race car, it isn't going to win any races. If you give your car the highest-octane fuel available, it's going to run like a champ. Your body is the same way. Food is your fuel. Give your body what it needs to run well, and you will get awesome sculpting results. Feed it the wrong fuel, and you'll get nowhere fast.

Carbohydrates

Carbohydrates should be the backbone of your body-sculpting nutrition. The _carbohydrate_ is the primary fuel source the body uses during high-intensity activity such as weight training, and the brain and nervous systems use it almost exclusively for energy. Lately, carbs have gotten a lot of bad press as being responsible for making people fat—hence all the low-carb fad diets outlined in Chapter 3. You now know that low-carb diets are not the answer and do not fit into a body-sculpting business plan, so you can feel comfortable about eating a high percentage of your daily calories from carbs. In fact, carbohydrates are often called the flame that burns fat because your body needs carbs to maintain the chemical processes that allow you to burn fat. When you run out of carbs, your body has to rely on protein to help burn fat; this is a really slow process that decreases your energy levels and diminishes your ability to exercise.

Trainer Talk _____

Carbohydrates come in three distinct types. Complex carbohydrates, a.k.a. starches, should make up the majority of your carbohydrate intake. Examples of these are whole grains, cereals, and vegetables. Simple sugars are those found naturally in milk products and fruit. Refined sugars (which you should avoid) are found in foods such as sodas, candy, and ice cream.

Carbohydrates are usually categorized as either starches or sugars, which are actually quite different. Starches, also called complex carbohydrates, are found in whole grains, cereals, vegetables, and dried beans and peas. Sugars are broken down into two more categories: simple and refined. Simple sugars are found naturally in milk products and fruit. Refined sugars, on the other hand, are manufactured and added to the foods you eat, usually in the form of sucrose and high-fructose corn syrup. Refined sugars make up a large part of sodas, fruit drinks, cookies, jam, candy, and ice cream. This is probably why carbohydrates have gotten a bad rap; if you eat a lot of foods with refined sugars, you will probably gain weight because you end up eating a lot of calories you don't burn off. Unfortunately, the refined sugars taste good! This doesn't mean that you shouldn't ever eat products with refined sugars. If you tried to exclude refined sugars from your diet completely, you would probably find yourself eliminating some of your favorite foods (especially the sweet stuff). Instead, try to eat more complex starch carbohydrates whenever possible, and save the refined sugars for special occasions and treats (this is explained in more detail in the next chapter).

The starches (complex carbs) are the foods our society has begun eating less of but needs to eat more of. Very few people eat fruits and vegetables every day, foods that contain complex carbs. In fact, a recent study of working adults found that the average person eats about half the necessary amount of starches and twice the amount of refined sugars.

So how many carbohydrates do you need? It depends. Most recommendations state that 55–70 percent of your total daily calories should come from carbohydrates, and that the majority of those should be from complex carbs (starches). It's pretty tough to have the same percentage of foods every day, so the range allows you to have more carbs some days and fewer carbs other days. You should get between 2.5 and 4.5 grams of carbohydrate for each pound you currently weigh. (Note that the number of carbs you need will decrease as you lose body-fat weight.) This number represents enough carbs to support your body-sculpting activities without having extra that can be stored as fat. For example, a 135-pound person would need to eat between 338 and 608 grams of carbs each day. On days when your activity level is higher, you should eat more carbs; on days when you don't exercise as much or are taking a day off, aim for the lower end of the range.

Proteins

Proteins are called the building blocks of the body because they are essential for muscle growth and for keeping all the body's systems working properly. However, high-protein diets do not make the body build muscle faster. Just as with carbohydrates, your body needs an optimal level of protein; any extra is stored as fat.

Protein is used for energy only if you have totally run out of carbohydrates. As I mentioned earlier, when you start relying on the calories from protein for energy, your body slows down. It takes a long time to turn protein calories into the type of energy your muscles need (you actually turn them into a form of carbohydrate), and that causes your body to slow down. Another reason you don't want to rely on protein for energy is that if your body has to burn protein for energy, it can't use it to build muscle tissue. One of your body-sculpting goals is to increase lean muscle tissue, so you want to be sure the protein you eat is being used for that purpose, not to get you through your workouts. After all, what's the point in exercising if your body doesn't have the protein you need to build muscle tissue? You basically end up spinning your wheels and exercising for nothing.

No Pain—Just Gain
Your body slows down when it begins to rely on protein for energy. This is why a high-protein/low-carb diet is not recommended to reach your body-sculpting goals. Your body burns carbohydrates much more efficiently, which leads to better body-sculpting results.

Because your protein calories mainly will be used for building lean tissue, you don't need a whole lot every day. Your protein intake should be between 12 and 15 percent of your total daily calories. This equals about 0.5 to 1 gram of protein for each pound you weigh. Our 135-pound person, therefore, would need 68 to 135 grams of protein each day. How much protein you eat each day does not depend on your activity level the way your carbohydrate intake does. You should try to eat the same amount of protein every day because your body is always working on building lean muscle tissue if you are doing body-sculpting exercises. When you aren't exercising (while you work, sleep, watch TV, or read this book), your muscles are recovering, which is when protein is needed the most, so strive to maintain adequate protein intake every day.

Protein is found in almost every type of food you can imagine. However, some foods, such as meats and eggs, are higher in protein; other foods, such as fruits, don't have much protein. Unfortunately, some foods that are good sources of protein often have a large amount of fat. Good sources of protein include red meat, chicken, fish, eggs, beans, and legumes.

Eating a variety of protein sources is also important because not all proteins are the same. Proteins are made up of a number of amino acids. A complete protein, found in foods such as eggs, has all the necessary amino acids. Other proteins, such as cereals, are incomplete because they don't have all the necessary amino acids. If you eat a variety of protein sources, you will be able to get all the necessary amino acids, and your body can build muscle tissue with ease.

Fat

Before we start, please note that not all fat is bad. Everyone requires some fat to keep the body working properly and aid tasks such as vitamin absorption and testosterone formation. The problem is that the typical American diet is 34 percent fat, which is much too high. Both the American Heart Association and the Subcommittee on Nutrition of the United Nations agree that fat should provide between 15 and 20 percent of your daily calories. For most people, just decreasing fat intake from 34 percent to 20 percent will cause a reduction in body fat because they will stop storing the excess. On the other hand, intakes of less than 10 percent have been shown to decrease testosterone production and muscle development, and decrease the body's ability to absorb vitamins A, D, E, and K. Even if you have some excess fat stored that you want to get rid of, you need fat in your diet. Your stored fat cannot help your body with vitamin absorption and other necessary processes. Only fat that is moving through the digestive process and through the bloodstream can do this.

Earlier I said that each gram of fat has 9 calories (more than twice as much as a gram of carb or protein). With so many calories in each gram of fat, you don't have to eat much fat to get to 15–20 percent of your calories. Unfortunately, the things we love to eat usually have a lot of fat grams and, therefore, a lot of calories in them. Nature's cruel trick is that fat provides much of food's flavor and texture.

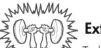

Extra Rep

To keep the body processing normally, fat should be an integral part of everyone's diet. Aim to eat 15–20 percent of your daily calories from fat. This will provide you with the fat your body needs, without excess your body will store as extra weight.

Fat also provides a lot of calories and is thus a great source of energy. However, this doesn't mean you should eat more fat when you need more energy. You already have fat stored in your body that needs to be burned, so don't eat any more than you need.

Vitamins and Minerals

Your body needs many other elements than the big three for optimum performance. Your body also needs vitamins and minerals. Perhaps you already take a daily multivitamin or antioxidant, or you supplement with iron or folic acid. Do you know why you do it? Vitamins and minerals are the microscopic elements that make all the chemical processes that occur in our bodies possible. Without vitamins and minerals, we can't do the things we need to, such as breathing, talking, and walking.

From 1941 to 1997, the Food and Nutrition Board of the National Academy of Sciences published the Recommended Daily Allowances (RDAs) for vitamins and minerals. The amount of each vitamin and mineral was determined based on what was needed to help a vitamin- and mineral-deficient individual return to normal levels. In 1997, the RDAs were changed to the Recommended Dietary Allowances, with an emphasis on long-term health instead of deficiency. When you look at a bottle of vitamins or minerals, you can see how much of the RDA each pill provides. A quick scan of the shelves at your local drugstore will show that you can buy pills that contain up to 5,000 percent of a certain vitamin or mineral RDA.

Unfortunately, too much of a good thing can also be bad. As science learns more about what certain vitamins and minerals do, the media push us to take more of them every day. I actually knew a man who couldn't eat breakfast because he got full just from taking his daily 20 vitamin and mineral supplements. If you are at the point that you have more pills to take than food to eat, something is wrong.

All your body requires is 100 percent of the recommended amount of vitamins and minerals; it expels any extra. Your body cannot store vitamins and minerals. Nor will taking more than 100 percent of the recommended amount make your body work any better. In fact, the Academy of Sciences has also published the levels at which certain vitamins and minerals can become dangerous. It's called a level of toxicity—the vitamin or mineral becomes toxic to the body. Eating a varied, balanced diet with the right percentages of each nutrient will usually provide you with 100 percent of all the vitamins and minerals you need. If you are not eating a variety of foods, but you get stuck in a rut eating the same things all the time, a multivitamin that provides 100 percent of all the vitamins and minerals can help you meet your nutritional goals. In fact, a multivitamin that provides only 100 percent of all the vitamins and minerals, but not more than 100 percent, is usually safe for everyone. (I strongly suggest you consult your doctor or an R.D. before taking any vitamin or mineral supplement, however, just to be sure.) A list of all the current RDAs is available in Appendix C.

No Pain—Just Gain

When it comes to vitamins and minerals, too much of a good thing can actually be dangerous. Avoid vitamins that provide much more than the 100 percent recommended daily levels. Too much of a certain vitamin or mineral can be toxic to your body.

Supplements

Dietary supplements have started to appear on grocery store shelves, in advertisements in your favorite magazines and newspapers, and now in specialty stores that sell only supplements. The key to keep in mind about dietary supplements is that they are what they claim to be: supplements. The word *supplement* means "in addition to." Supplements should never take the place of the carbohydrates, protein, and fat you get from regular food. However, they can help you get enough nutrients on days when you are extra busy, when you need a quick good-for-you snack, or when you are traveling and cannot cook for yourself.

Supplement manufacturers would have you believe you can't possibly shape the body you want with regular food and that their product has something special that will sculpt a better body than that of your normal food–eating friends. These claims couldn't be further from the truth. Supplements can help you reach your goals, but they can't do it by themselves. Food will always be your best fuel, but if you find that you are having problems getting enough food to meet the demands of your body-sculpting business plan, supplements can help.

That being said, the most helpful dietary supplements are those that provide calories in proportion to your regular eating habits. If you are trying to maintain a diet of 70 percent carbs, 15 percent fat, and 15 percent protein, look for calorie supplements that have about the same proportions. Most of the time, the serving size of a supplement is close to that of a small meal or a large snack. These "meal replacements," as they are usually called, can provide you with good sources of nutrients and some of the vitamins and minerals you need. Examples are Slimfast shakes, SuperShake, Ensure, and even Carnation Instant Breakfast Drink. Even though the commercials say it's okay to "have one for breakfast, one for lunch, and then eat a sensible dinner," you shouldn't rely on supplements because they do not have all the qualities of regular food—qualities such as taste, variety, texture, and taste. (Yes, I said *taste* twice.)

Besides drink form, supplements are appearing more frequently as "energy bars" or "meal bars." Like their liquid counterparts, they are good for a little something extra but should not be regularly substituted for normal food. Supplements do not provide all the necessary naturally occurring vitamins and minerals that foods do. Anything in a supplement has been chemically made, altered, or enhanced, which is not always a good thing.

Many supplements also have absolutely no value. Manufacturers have taken to marketing obscure herbs with "secret" ingredients that claim to solve all your problems. For instance, Horny Goat Weed, Yohimbe Bark, Noni Juice, and Octacosanol are all supposed to help your body become more wonderful than ever, with just three pills a day for six months (which will cost you a few hundred dollars). But there isn't any real scientific proof that any of it works.

What Are You Drinking?

Have you ever sat down to a meal without something to drink? Probably not. When you go to the grocery store, you find entire aisles devoted to beverages of some form. Whether it's plain old water, sodas, fruit juices, or even alcoholic drinks, there are tons of options to quench your thirst. The downside to this plethora of fluids is that you have to make another decision: What should you be drinking?

The human body is comprised of more than 75 percent water. Your muscles are mostly water, and even your fat has water. Clearly, water is extremely important. Does this mean you should drink only plain water?

Thankfully, it doesn't. The main ingredient in all drinks is water, so no matter what you drink, you'll be getting the benefits of water. That said, it's important to note that plain old water is still the best thing for your body, simply because many of the other choices have additional "empty" calories and chemicals we can't pronounce, and some can actually cause dehydration.

Fluids should serve one main purpose: to keep you hydrated. During hot and humid days, water is essential for survival. When you are in the middle of your body-sculpting workout and get thirsty, water will quench your thirst faster than anything on the market. Sports drinks such as Gatorade and Powerade also help quench your thirst and provide you with replacement electrolytes and extra energy, but water has always been shown to be the most effective fluid for preventing dehydration.

Dehydration is really a lot more than just being thirsty. Your muscles are mostly water, so losing that water impairs your exercise performance—you won't be able to complete your body-sculpting workout. Additionally, if you lose 1 percent or more of your body weight through dehydration (figure this amount as: body weight × 0.01), your core temperature increases, which can lead to heat exhaustion, heat stroke, and even death. For a 150-pound person, a 1.5-pound drop in body weight from heavy sweating during a workout could cause heat exhaustion.

If you do choose to drink sports drinks, soda, or any other fluid with additional calories, be sure to account for these in your daily nutritional plan. I have seen numerous clients cut many calories simply by eliminating sodas, which can have as many as 150 calories per 12-ounce serving. Finally, alcoholic beverages can act as a dehydrator by causing you to use the bathroom more frequently; plus, they usually have quite a few calories.

The Least You Need to Know

- A calorie is simply a unit of energy; your body needs calories to keep functioning.

- Carbohydrates are not the enemy (neither are proteins or fats). Taken in the right balance, the body needs them to function normally.

- Try to get the majority of your carbohydrates from complex carbohydrates (veggies, beans, and whole-grain foods) rather than from refined sugars (white bread and pasta, jams, and sodas).

- Proteins should make up approximately 12–15 percent of your total daily calories. Relying on protein for the majority of your calories will slow you down and burn calories less efficiently, hindering your body-sculpting goals.

- Fats are a necessary part of everyone's diet to aid in the absorption of vitamins and other vital functions.

- Don't forget to hydrate your body! Water is the best hydrator, but sport drinks are also an efficient way to replace much-need fluids while pursuing your body-sculpting goals.

In This Chapter

- ◆ Determining your ideal number of daily calories
- ◆ Following the food pyramid to body-sculpting success
- ◆ Tips on balancing breakfast, lunch, dinner, and snacks
- ◆ Reading food labels properly
- ◆ Strategies for dining out

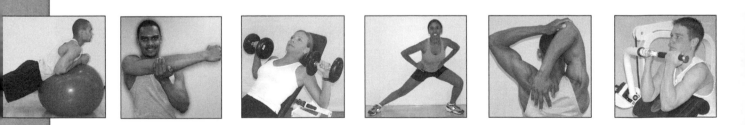

Chapter 6

Reality Eating

In the last chapter, you learned the differences among carbohydrates, fats, proteins, vitamins, and minerals, and what each of them will and won't do for a body-sculpting business plan. This chapter brings together these basics to give you an understanding of how to eat in real life.

Most diet books and fad diet plans are nearly impossible to follow for any length of time because they assume you live in a perfect world—a bubble that contains only the few foods you are allowed to eat. Of course, real life presents new and different situations daily that may not befit a perfect eating regimen. This chapter prepares you to face these daily challenges, to help you come out well fed *and* well sculpted.

How Many Calories?

Chapter 5 outlined the optimum nutrition breakdown for your total calorie intake: 55–70 percent from carbohydrates, 12–15 percent from protein, and 15–20 percent from fat sources. Yes, contrary to much of the current fad diet thinking, your diet should actually consist mostly of carbohydrates, with some fat and some protein to balance it out. High-carb diets are not evil (see Chapter 5).

More important are the total calories you eat every day. Unfortunately, this isn't always the easiest number to figure out. Lots of formulas and tables attempt to pin down the ideal number, given your height and weight, but they all fall short. The problem with the formulas you often see in books and on the Internet is that they don't take into account how many calories you burn every day. Remember, successful body sculpting involves finding the right balance of calories *in* versus calories *out*. It's easy for me to simply advise you to eat 1,500 calories a day to lose body fat, but if you burn only 1,400 calories a day, you'll just end up gaining fat. This is why it's critical to estimate how many calories per day you burn as closely as possible.

Unfortunately, there's no magic formula to figure this out. One thing science has determined is that nobody should consume less than 1,200 calories a day, which is what the body requires to stay alive and maintain proper functions. Beyond that, we have to make some educated guesses. Each of us burns different amounts of calories each day, and no two days are the same (which is why we won't eat the same every day). The key is balancing your food intake with your activity level. On days when you do longer, more intense workouts, you'll be able to eat more. On days when you rest and don't work out, you don't need to eat as much. It's all about balance.

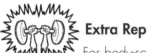

Extra Rep

For body-sculpting success, the ideal breakdown of your daily calories should consist of 55–70 percent carbohydrates, 12–15 percent protein, and 15–20 percent fat.

The only true way for you to determine how many daily calories you really require is to chart both your food and beverage intake, your exercise levels, and your body weight or body fat. Over time, you will notice one of three trends:

◆ You are gaining weight and fat, which means you're eating too much.

◆ You're maintaining your weight without gain or loss, which means you're eating as much as you burn.

◆ You're losing weight and body fat, which means you're burning more calories than you ingest.

It's nearly impossible to accurately change your daily eating habits based on that day's activity level, so I recommend that you take a slightly longer-term strategy. This is where keeping a journal really pays off. Monitor your progress weekly and monthly. If you notice a change on the scale and in your body composition (fat percentage), refer to your journal to analyze your eating and activity behavior. Identify what helped you (cutting 100 calories per day, perhaps, or adding 15 minutes of daily cardio training) or hurt you (extra servings at dinner, skipping too many workouts this week). Then simply reinforce the behaviors that brought you success, and change those that didn't quite get you there.

For now, because you're just starting out, think back over the last couple months. Has your body been through any changes—weight gain or weight loss? Or have you simply maintained the same weight and body composition? This can provide you with a good starting point. In fact, unless you've been gaining weight, a good strategy for beginning your sculpting program is to keep eating the same number of calories you do now, but change the percentages as outlined at the beginning of this chapter: 55–70 percent carbs, 12–15 percent protein, and 15–20 percent fat.

No Pain—Just Gain

Don't rely on formulas alone to figure out your optimum daily calorie intake. Keep a detailed journal so that, over time, you can compare your daily calories and activity level to your actual results. If you've lost weight and gained muscle, keep doing what you're doing; if you're not getting results, reduce your calories or increase activity.

A Pyramid of Food

So you've committed to adjusting your diet to include our recommended nutrition ratio of carbs to proteins to fat. Even before you figure out your ideal calorie intake, you'll want to be aware of what foods fall into which categories. Using the USDA *food pyramid* is probably the simplest way to figure this out. The pyramid is based on a simple concept: We need more of the foods at the foundation of the pyramid (carbs) and less of the foods at the top of the pyramid (proteins and fats).

Trainer Talk _____

The **food pyramid** is the USDA's recommendations for eating a healthful diet. We recommend it highly for a nutrition plan that will help you achieve your body-sculpting goals.

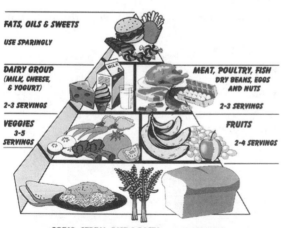

FATS, OILS & SWEETS
USE SPARINGLY

DAIRY GROUP
(MILK, CHEESE,
& YOGURT)
2-3 SERVINGS

MEAT, POULTRY, FISH
DRY BEANS, EGGS
AND NUTS
2-3 SERVINGS

VEGGIES
3-5 SERVINGS

FRUITS
2-4 SERVINGS

BREAD, CEREAL, RICE & PASTA   6-11 SERVINGS

Because it is such a simple guide, the food pyramid has received some criticism in the past. Although it may not be a perfect system, and we generally follow it in a less-than-perfect way, it does provide a valuable and accurate nutrition structure to help achieve body-sculpting goals.

The food pyramid accurately reflects our recommended carb/protein fat ratio. The bottom two levels, made up of bread, cereal, rice, pasta, vegetables, and fruits, are all carbohydrates. The next highest level contains foods with more protein and fat. The very top includes the high-fat foods we don't need a lot of. Note that "don't need a lot of" does *not* mean "never eat." With the pyramid—and the eating plan I recommend—nothing is excluded. You can eat a large variety of foods; you just need to control the amounts.

You can control these amounts by paying attention to serving sizes, which are also outlined on the pyramid. I've heard complaints that there is no way you can eat the pyramid's recommended servings without gaining weight. In reality, you can. The most important factor to understand is how much food actually constitutes a serving size. It's not that platter-size plate you get at a restaurant; it's not even a regular-size plate you might use at home. Instead, here are some examples of what constitutes a serving size for each of the food groups:

◆ **Bread, cereal, rice, and pasta.** 1 slice of bread; 1 ounce of cereal; ½ cup cooked cereal, rice, pasta, or grits

◆ **Fruit group.** 1 whole apple, orange, pear, banana, etc; ¾ cup juice; 1 melon wedge; ½ grapefruit; ½ cup cooked or canned fruit

◆ **Vegetable group.** ½ cup cooked vegetable, 1 cup chopped raw vegetable, 1 cup leafy raw vegetable, ½ cup cooked beans, ¾ cup vegetable juice

◆ **Meat, poultry, fish, eggs, and nuts.** 2–3 ounces cooked lean meat, fish, or poultry; ⅓ cup nuts; ½ cup tofu; 1–2 egg whites; ½ cup cooked beans or peas; 2 tablespoons peanut butter

◆ **Milk, yogurt, and cheese.** 1 cup low-fat milk or yogurt, 2 ounces processed cheese, 1½ ounces low-fat cheese

◆ **Fats, oils, and sweets.** 1 teaspoon spreads, vegetable oils, or butter; 1 tablespoon dressing

> **Extra Rep**
> The key to proper nutrition lies not just in what you eat, but also how much you eat. Follow the food pyramid's serving size guidelines to help you determine the proper quantities of food to consume.

Simply follow the food source ratio indicated on the food pyramid, along with the recommended servings. On less active days, keep servings at the recommended minimum; on more active days, treat yourself to the upper end of recommended servings.

Time to Eat

Now that you understand what to eat and how much to eat, let's discuss when to eat it. I like to think of the body as a car and your food as the fuel. You have to put fuel in your car before it will go anywhere, and you have to keep re-fueling it for it to continue running. Our bodies are the same: We need food to get moving and to keep moving. The problem is, because our society has grown accustomed to the idea of three square meals a day, we often eat too little when we need more, and too much when we need less. Using the "your body is a car" analogy, think of it like this: You put gas in your car when you need to go somewhere, not when you're going to stay parked. Your body works the same way: It needs more fuel when you want it to move and less when you'll be relatively immobile.

The other choice is to eat whenever you want and just store any excess calories to use later—except that you are going to store them as fat, and that makes it harder to burn off later.

Breakfast Basics

Breakfast is the most important meal of the day. Ever heard that? Despite this adage, today's reality is more like "Breakfast is the most skipped meal of the day." Too many people skip breakfast because they don't feel hungry or they don't make the time to eat. But just as you wouldn't try to drive your car on an empty gas tank, you shouldn't deprive your body of fuel.

The advice to eat a good breakfast is based on simple body chemistry discussed in Chapter 5. The body needs carbs to burn fat. If it doesn't have carbs readily available, it has to turn to protein to get the fat-burning fires going. Because you don't store excess protein, the body must use protein from your lean tissues: your muscles. So basically, you end up burning muscle tissue for energy because you didn't take time for breakfast. And all your hard work to build that muscle is set back.

> **No Pain—Just Gain**
> Never skip breakfast. You may think you're "saving" calories, but you'll be slowing down your body-sculpting goals because of the way your body chemistry works.

Here's another way to think of it: You've just slept for the last eight or so hours—without eating. How often do you go eight hours during the day without a meal or snack? When you wake up, you've just finished an eight-hour fast, and your body needs fuel—energy from food.

Even if you don't feel hungry, your muscles don't have the proper fuel to burn. So at that point, you need to separate the "feeling" of your stomach being empty from your body's need for fuel. You may not feel hungry, but you really are; it's just that your stomach isn't sending you that signal.

Breakfast, like all your meals, should be a proportional mix of carbohydrates, protein, and fat. Your body requires all of them to work at its best until lunch. If you eat at least one serving from each of the food groups on the pyramid, it should fill you up. Unfortunately, eating a small "breakfast bar" or some sort of "breakfast drink" usually doesn't provide the number of calories you need to get you through the morning.

Power Lunch

Lunch is decidedly the second most important meal of the day. Unfortunately, many times lunch becomes a quick and easy feeding frenzy. The pressures of work may give you only 30 minutes (or less) to find, fix, and eat lunch. As a result, many people skip lunch, eat only a small snack, or rush through a fast-food drive-thru for the sake of convenience. But lunch should be taken more seriously because it's the meal that fuels you for the longest and usually busiest part of your day. During the approximately six hours between lunch and dinner (noon to 6 P.M.), we finish our work day, run errands, work out, and get home to finish chores. For all this, you need some serious fuel.

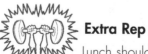

Extra Rep

Lunch should be the largest meal of your day, with a healthful balance of carbs, proteins, and fat.

Based on these facts, lunch should be the biggest meal of the day, from which you should get the majority of your daily calories. Like breakfast, a good lunch should balance carbohydrates, proteins, and fat, with a few more servings than breakfast to satisfy you. If you're always rushed at lunch, take some time to pre-plan and pack a healthful meal so you won't fall into the trap of skipping this meal or eating fast food.

Rethinking Dinner

For almost all Americans, dinner has become the biggest meal of the day. Our thinking is that dinner should include a lot of servings of meat and potatoes and veggies and bread, and, of course, dessert. Yet for the majority of my clients, just changing their approach to dinner has catapulted their body-sculpting nutrition to a new level. Breaking away from your old notions of dinner will help you, too.

Q&A

Is it true that I shouldn't eat late in the evening?

Yes. You should consume the majority of your daily calories early in the day so you have the time and activity levels to burn them off before bed. Any excess calories will only be stored as fat.

The lapse between dinner and bedtime is relatively short. If you eat dinner around 6 or 7 and go to bed around 10 or 11, that leaves only about 4 or 5 hours for you to digest and burn all those dinner calories. The average time it takes to digest a big meal is two to three hours. Until the food is digested and the nutrients are absorbed into the bloodstream, you can't use those calories. For instance, that walk right after dinner won't burn the calories you just consumed. In addition, the time between dinner and bedtime is usually filled with lower-energy activities—watching TV, doing household chores, talking on the phone. These activities do not require many calories. So the result of eating that big meal is that the excess, unburned calories are stored as fat.

The solution is simple: a smaller dinner. Eat just enough so you're satiated—but not bursting at the seams. Eat what you can burn so nothing is left to store as fat. If you work out during the evening after dinner, you can afford to eat a bit more; if you're completely sedentary after dinner, eat less.

Savvy Snacks

I am a big proponent of snacks—the right snacks, that is. Snacking is great, as long as you're eating something you will burn off. Unfortunately, most of what we consider snack foods are really high in fat, such as candy bars, snack cakes, and potato chips. But by rethinking what we view as snacks, we have a great opportunity to catch up on the areas of the food pyramid in which we're lacking—usually fruits and vegetables. These foods, which are high in carbohydrates, have a little protein, have no fat, will boost your blood sugar level, give your muscles energy, and carry you through to the next meal.

A lot of controversy has arisen over "high-carb" snacks that raise your blood sugar, cause a spike in your insulin levels, and supposedly cause the carbs to be stored as fat (this is where the low-carb diets get their ideas). It is true that a high-carbohydrate food will raise your blood sugar—in fact, anytime you eat anything, your blood sugar rises. It is also true that your insulin levels will spike. Insulin causes the sugar to enter the cells, where it can be used for energy.

People who don't get this boost in insulin in response to eating are labeled diabetic. So insulin is good. Finally, the only way carbs get stored as fat is if they are not used. If you eat and sit, they will be stored as fat (probably on your hips and butt), but if you move, you will burn them.

The danger of snacking is that we often do it not because we're hungry, but because we're bored, tired, or nervous. "Good" snacking should occur only when we're actually hungry, to tide us over between meals. If you feel you've burned all the food and calories from your last meal, a 100- to 200-calorie snack will provide enough energy to keep you going for a good hour and a half.

Shopping for Labels

Finding the foods to fit into your body-sculpting food pyramid is as easy as reading the label. The problem is, the labels on most foods aren't always easy to read until you know exactly what to look for.

A few years ago, new laws were passed to regulate the information included on food labels. The result is more complete, consistent, and helpful nutritional information that provides you with an accurate summary of what's inside the package. This information includes the following:

◆ The serving size
◆ How many servings are in the container
◆ The number of calories per serving
◆ How many of those calories are from fat
◆ The total grams of fat, carbohydrate, and protein
◆ The percent of RDA for certain vitamins

Extra Rep

For certain food items that are meant to be mixed with other ingredients before you eat them—such as a cake mix that requires milk, eggs, and oil—you will find a second column that shows the carb, fat, and protein information when mixed with the extra ingredients.

Nutrition Facts

Serving Size 1 piece
Servings Per Container 6

Amount Per Serving
Calories 130   Calories from Fat 45

	% Daily Value*
Total Fat 5g	8%
Saturated Fat 2g	9%
Cholesterol 15mg	5%
Potassium 45mg	1%
Sodium 210mg	9%
Total Carbohydrate 21g	7%
Sugars 11g	
Protein 2g	
Iron	4%
Thiamin	4%
Riboflavin	4%
Niacin	2%
Folic Acid	4%

Not a significant source of dietary fiber, vitamin A, vitamin C and calcium.

*Percent Daily Values are based on a 2,000 calorie diet. Your values may be higher or lower depending on your calorie needs.

A food label has information you can use to decide whether a food is a wise choice for your body business plan.

When referring to a food label, look first for the number of calories and then the number of calories derived from fat. If a food has a fat percentage that's too high, it's best to avoid it. Con-sider this example: A food label says each serving provides 137 calories, and 45 of them are from fat. The label also says that a serving contains 5 grams of fat, 2 grams of protein, and 21 grams of carbohydrates. At a quick glance, it might seem that this food is high in carbs and low in fat and protein, but remember that each gram of fat has more than twice the calories of a gram of carbs or protein. In reality, this food gets 33 percent of its calories from fat (45 ÷ 137). This is not a balanced food you want in your body-sculpting nutrition program.

Also look at the number of servings per container. Many small foods that are typically eaten completely in one sitting are actually labeled as more than one serving. For instance, some candy bars—which we tend to eat all at once—are listed as two or three servings per bar. If you thought you were getting a snack with only 130 calories, but you didn't notice it contained 3 servings (with each serving being 130 calories), you may have eaten 390 calories by mistake. A manufacturer can divide a high-fat and high-calorie food into several servings to make it seem like a good thing.

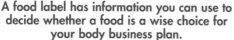

Extra Rep

Try to choose foods that are made up of 20 percent fat or less. To figure this out, divide the number of calories from fat by the total number of calories on any given food label.

As you wander through the grocery store, you may be drawn to foods that advertise themselves as low fat, low calorie, light, or fat free. However, your definition of those terms may not be what the manufacturer had in mind. When the label laws were changed, certain terms manufacturers had been using in misleading ways were given strict definitions. Here are some of the most common ones:

◆ A "low-fat" food has 3 grams of fat or less.

◆ A food that is "low in saturated fat" contains 1 gram or less of saturated fat.

- A "low-calorie" food has 40 calories or less per serving.
- A "lean" meat or poultry product must contain less than 10 grams of fat and 4.5 grams or less of saturated fat.
- "Reduced" means the food has been nutritionally altered from its original state—not necessarily good for you.
- The term "less" does not have to refer to calories; it can mean that the food is presented in a lighter way.
- "Light" or "lite" means that a product has been altered to contain one-third fewer calories or half the fat of the original food—again, not necessarily good for you.
- "Free" means that the products has "virtually" no fat, but serving sizes can be manipulated to keep the serving size so small that there is very little fat in it.
- "Calorie-free" foods have 5 calories or less per serving.

Take the time to read the labels on foods before you buy them. It may take a while to get the hang of it, but before long, you will be cruising through the grocery store knowing exactly which choices are healthful and which are not.

Dining Out and Eating on the Go

In an ideal world, we shop for and cook all our own food so that we have total control over what goes in our bodies. In the real world, we often eat at restaurants and order takeout. It is possible to manipulate your nutrition plan to include eating out and getting the occasional drive-thru fast-food fix. However, it's nearly impossible to eat all your meals out and expect to meet your body-sculpting goals.

Unfortunately, food served in restaurants and fast-food establishments is not normally designed to reflect the food pyramid. In fact, you'll get a more accurate representation of what most restaurants serve if you flip the food pyramid upside down: a lot of fat and very few carbohydrates. I believe it's no coincidence that as the number of restaurants and fast-food places has increased in this country, so has the number of overweight and obese people.

With that said, to eat out and stay on your body-sculpting regimen, you have to plan ahead. Choose restaurants that you know have low-fat, healthful choices on the menu. Stay away from fried foods (no food is good for you after it's been soaked in oil that's 100 percent fat), heavy dressings, and cream sauces. Look for lean cuts of meat, poultry, and fish (without cream or butter sauces); pasta with red sauce; steamed vegetables; and fruit for dessert. Beware of "good for you" salad bars that have plenty of good veggies and ingredients, with heavy, fat-filled dressings to fatten them right up.

Don't be afraid to ask for items that aren't on the menu. I regularly ask for a vegetable plate (baked potato with low-fat or fat-free dressing instead of butter and sour cream, and steamed veggie of the day), chicken without skin, bread not brushed with butter, and pasta not tossed in oil. Restaurants will be happy to provide you with more healthful alternatives if they think you will be a return customer.

Another trick that I like to use at restaurants is to split the meal in half—half for now, half for later. The size of serving plates at restaurants has gotten totally out of control. Instead of a plate, you get a platter. It's usually much more than a normal person needs at one meal, so split it up. Ask for a to-go box before you even begin eating. Then you have lunch for tomorrow all wrapped up and ready to go—without being tempted to clean your plate.

Most fast-food places now offer more healthful alternatives to their staple items. Burger places usually have a grilled chicken sandwich, and fish places offer baked fish instead of fried fish. Even so, it's nearly impossible to get a balanced meal at a fast-food place, so avoid them unless it's absolutely necessary. The nutritional information of most popular fast-food restaurants is available on their websites, or they will give it to you if you go in and ask (just don't supersize while you're there).

Extra Rep

Almost all restaurants serve much more food than you require. To avoid overeating, take home half of what's on your plate and avoid supersizing when at fast-food restaurants.

Planning and Putting It All Together

Now that you have a good idea of how you should eat, when you should eat, and where you should eat, it's time to make a plan. Just as you have a solid exercise plan, you need a solid nutrition plan. With your car, you can stop at any old gas station whenever you need fuel, and the gas is always the same. That's not so with your body. Sit down at the beginning of each week, make a grocery list, and go shopping. Cook several days' worth of food at one time, and freeze individual servings until it's time to eat.

You may not always know what you want to eat in advance—and we all get cravings now and then. What separates the flabby from the sculpted is what you do when faced with that craving. Have an action plan ready: "The next

time I feel like getting a burger and fries, I'll go to the deli and have a lean roast-beef sandwich and a bowl of fruit instead." If you have a plan, you won't get caught up in the moment and get pulled away from your goals.

Eating properly takes time and practice. I tell every one of my clients to make incremental changes. Start with one big thing that you can do to make your nutrition better right now: Maybe pack your lunches instead of eating fast food, or replace that daily chocolate bar with a piece of fruit. Work on that one thing until you've developed a new habit and then go after the next one thing. Don't try to change your nutrition overnight; your body will rebel, and the cravings will be uncontrollable. Slowly change for the better, and your body will adapt without any problem—and the results will show in the mirror.

The Least You Need to Know

- ◆ Journal your calorie intake, calories burned through activity, and weight; this will provide you with a benchmark with which to determine your ideal number of calories per day.
- ◆ Follow the food pyramid to determine the number of carb, protein, and fat servings you should have per day.
- ◆ Never skip breakfast.
- ◆ Make lunch your biggest meal of the day.
- ◆ Snacking is a great way to avoid over-indulging during your next meal, and be sure to choose snacks that have the right balance of carbs, protein, and fat.
- ◆ Read food labels carefully to make healthful choices when shopping and cooking.
- ◆ When eating out, eat only half your portion; most restaurants offer twice the amount of food you need.

In This Part

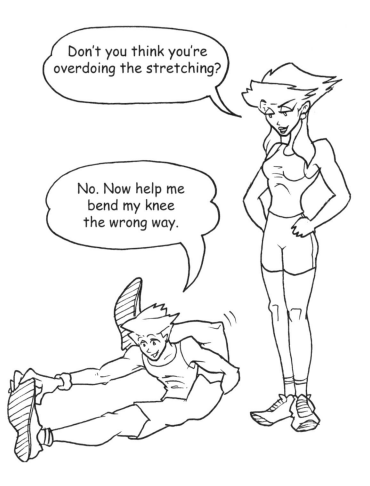

Part 3

The Building Blocks of Body Sculpting

Without bricks and mortar, you'll never get off the ground. Similarly, without stretching and aerobics, you'll have a tough time making any progress in your workouts. That's because both these components are the building blocks of your body-sculpting program, vital resources to help you strive toward a higher goal. Through stretching, you'll gain the flexibility you need to maximize your resistance training. Through aerobic activity, you'll burn that extra layer of fat to reveal the sculpted physique within. Part 3 provides you with all the instruction you need to shape your own bricks and mortar into the work of art you envision.

In This Chapter

◆ Why flexibility is important for body sculpting

◆ When to stretch

◆ Which muscles you need to stretch

◆ Simple stretching exercises for every muscle group

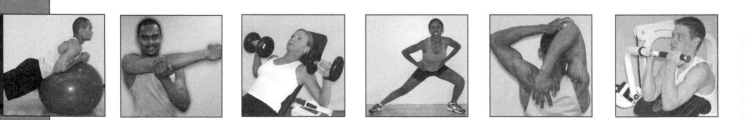

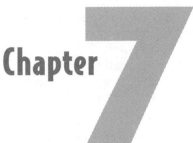

Chapter **7**

Stretch with Ease

Flexibility isn't about being able to put your foot behind your head (not something I recommend) or touch your toes. Flexibility is about moving freely, loosening up your muscles and joints, preventing injury, and helping you relax after a hard workout. Of all the elements of your body-sculpting program, stretching and flexibility training are the easiest. Although becoming more flexible won't be visible in the mirror, it will help you move better through your exercises and recover faster after your workouts, leaving you feeling strong instead of sore.

Flexibility Facts

Each of your joints has a natural range of motion in which movements are relatively easy. Unfortunately, as we age and our lives become more sedentary, we don't use that range of motion, so our bodies tighten up. It's another classic case of "use it or lose it." Injuries such as strains and sprains are often the result of forcing the body to move in a range of motion that it simply is no longer capable of. In fact, many chiropractors and orthopedic doctors agree that a great number of the injuries they treat could have been prevented if an individual was only more flexible. *Flexibility* is the secret behind gymnasts' incredible athletic maneuvers. It is also why, as we age, it becomes more difficult to do a split, even if you were once head cheerleader.

Trainer Talk ⎯⎯⎯⎯⎯⎯⎯⎯

Flexibility describes the comfortable range of motion your joints can move within. As we age and don't regularly move within that range of motion, our joints become "tight" and we lose our flexibility.

The good news is that even if you've lost flexibility, a regular regimen of simple stretching exercises will bring back your body's natural range of motion. By increasing your range of motion in each joint, you'll move more freely, more easily, and without pain. Think of the feeling you have when you first wake up in the morning: Your joints are tight and bound up. Now think of the feeling you get after you stretch and walk: Everything feels better! Flexibility training can give you that just-stretched feeling all the time.

Most important for our purposes, flexibility training will help you with your body-sculpting resistance training. If your joints are too tight to move through an exercise, you won't get the full benefit of that exercise. Greater flexibility will allow your muscles to do their job without fighting against tight joints, resulting in an easier workout and more sculpted muscles.

Finally, another valuable benefit of stretching and flexibility training is reduced stress and tension in your body. You contract and relax your muscles all day long, and they eventually need a break. Stretching helps you return your muscles to their natural resting length, which releases tension, prepares you for your next workout, and can help keep you from getting sore after resistance and aerobic activity.

Prestretch Warm-Up

Most muscle injuries occur when an individual's muscles are "cold"—that is, when they haven't been properly warmed up. To illustrate this, consider a piece of chewing gum. If the gum is cold and you try to bend it, it just breaks in two. When the gum is warm, it bends and stretches easily. Your muscles are the same way: When they are warm, they stretch; when they're cold, they tear. So you need to warm up your muscles before you stretch.

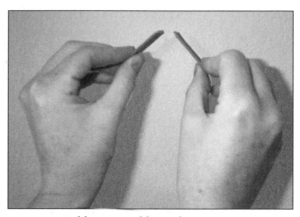

Cold gum = cold muscles = tears.

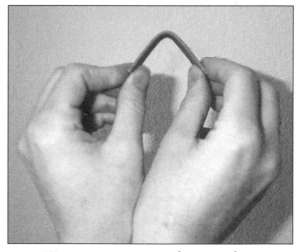

Warm gum = warm muscles = stretches.

No Pain—Just Gain

Even stretching requires a warm-up. Before you do your stretching exercises, be sure to do a few simple moves, such as walking or light repetitions, to ensure that your muscles are not "cold" and susceptible to injury.

A prestretch warm-up is as simple as walking around and moving your muscles and joints before you stretch them. By doing so, you'll become more flexible in less time.

Timing Is Everything

If the goal of stretching is to reduce the tension that's built up during your workout, prepare you for the next workout, and help prevent soreness after a workout, it makes sense that your flexibility training should always be done after exercise. You can fit flexibility training into your workout in two ways:

◆ Save all your stretching—for all parts of your body—until the end of your entire workout.

◆ Stretch each specific muscle immediately after you finish your body-sculpting exercise for that muscle.

Either way is fine. The important thing is to remember to do it.

How Long Does It Take?

Not only is stretching the easiest part of your body-sculpting routine, but it also takes the least amount of time. Each stretch should last approximately 15–30 seconds, depending on how flexible you are to begin with. If you are really tight and you really feel these stretches, start with 15 seconds per muscle group. As you loosen up, add more time. You should see more flexibility within a matter of days.

Repeat each stretch until you've accumulated one minute of stretch for each muscle group. So if you stretch 15 seconds, do it 4 times. If you stretch 30 seconds, do it twice. An entire stretching program that targets each muscle group in your body—for example, doing each of the stretches in this chapter for one minute each—will take less than 15 minutes.

Do I Have to Stretch All My Muscles?

You don't have to stretch all your muscles every time you work out; just focus on the ones you've worked that day. Because you have to warm up a muscle before you can stretch it, it makes sense that you don't stretch the muscles that you don't use.

Long-Necks

Even though we're not working neck muscles specifically, it's important to stretch the neck. That's because so many of the shoulder, back, and chest muscles you will work are attached to the joints of your neck.

For best results, do both of these neck stretches. You'll notice that these exercises work only the sides and back of the neck. When you stretch the sides, you also stretch the muscles in the front of your neck.

If you have had a neck injury or are experiencing any pain in your neck (and I'm not talking about your spouse or children), see a doctor or chiropractor before doing this stretch.

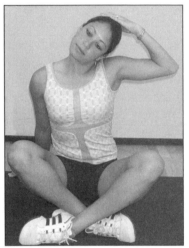

2. Use your hand to pull your head to the side until you feel a stretch on the other side of your neck.

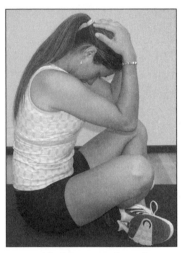

4. When your chin hits your chest, lean your upper body forward to increase the stretch.

Side Stretch

1. Sit on the floor or in a chair. You don't have to keep your back straight; in fact, you will get more stretch if you relax all your back muscles and "slump" forward a little.

2. Place one hand on the floor or on the chair seat and the other hand on top of your head. Let your head relax toward your shoulder, using your hand to pull your head down until you feel the stretch on the other side of your neck (the side of your resting hand). To make the stretch a little more intense, push the hand that is on the floor or chair seat down and away from you. Hold for 15–30 seconds and then repeat the stretch on the other side, moving from side to side until you get one minute of stretching on each side.

Back Stretch

3. Sitting in the same position as with the side stretch, place both hands on the top part of your head, slightly toward the back (see the photo for clarification). Your elbows should be pointed down in front of you.

4. Drop your chin toward your chest, and pull forward and down with both hands. When your chin comes in contact with your chest, lean your upper body forward, kind of like curling into a little ball, to increase the stretch. Hold for 15–30 seconds, and repeat as necessary to get one full minute of stretch.

Pectoral Twist

Although this exercise is called a pectoral twist, you'll generally feel these stretches more in your shoulder area than in your chest. That's because the chest muscles attach to your arms at the shoulder, so your joints are located there. You may not feel the stretching "burn" as with other stretches, but fear not: You're still getting results.

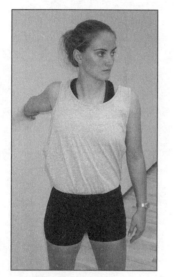

Turn your upper body away from your hand, as if you're looking back over your shoulder.

1. Stand about a foot away from a wall, a pole, or a tall piece of exercise equipment—something that you can grab hold of. Place your feet shoulder width apart for good balance. Reach one hand behind you and place it on the wall or whatever you are standing next to.
2. Keeping your arm straight, turn your shoulders away from the wall. Turn your upper body away from your hand, almost as if you're looking back over your other shoulder. Hold the stretch for 15–30 seconds; then switch to the other arm and stretch it for 15–30 seconds. Repeat the stretch on each arm until you've had a full minute of stretch.

Shoulder Squeeze

Whereas the previous exercise—the pectoral twist—stretches the front half of the shoulder, this exercise stretches the back half of the shoulder. Be sure to do both stretches to ensure that your shoulders stay loose and injury free.

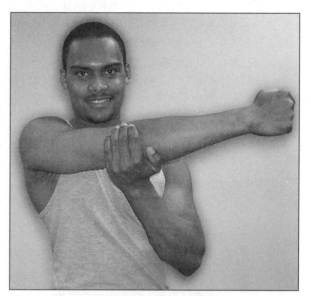

If you have trouble feeling the stretch, try to raise your arm higher under your chin.

1. Reach across your chest with one arm, and grasp that arm's elbow with your other hand. Hold your arm straight, keeping it just under your chin.
2. Use the hand on your elbow to push the arm against the chest. You should feel the stretch across the back of your shoulder. If you don't feel much stretch, raise your arm under your chin a little more. Hold the stretch for 15–30 seconds and then stretch the other arm. Alternate arms until you have completed one minute on each arm.

Bicep Push

Stretching the biceps is often overlooked, possibly because you don't feel the same amount of stretch as you do with other flexibility exercises. However, stretching the biceps is still important for preventing muscle strains and soreness after a workout.

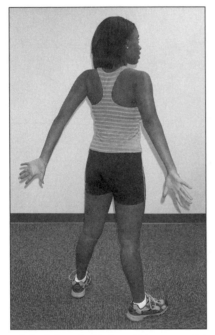

Push both hands back as far as possible.

1. Stand with your feet apart, hands down at your sides, and palms facing back behind you.
2. Keeping your arms straight, push both hands back as far as possible. You should feel a slight stretch at the elbow and down the front of your arm (the biceps). Hold for 15–30 seconds and then repeat until you finish a full minute.

Triceps Pretzel

Even if you don't do isolated triceps training, you still work the triceps during many chest and shoulder press exercises. So be sure to stretch these muscles after working the upper body. Not only is it good for you, but it also feels great.

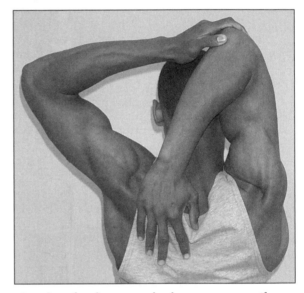

Reach as far down your back as you can, as if you were trying to scratch it.

1. Reach up and over your head with one hand. Pretend you are trying to scratch your back between your shoulder blades. Use the other hand to grasp the elbow that's up in the air.
2. Reach as far down your back as you can and then pull on your elbow with your other hand to increase the stretch a little more. Hold the stretch for 15–30 seconds, stretch the other arm, and repeat until both arms have had a minute of stretch each.

Hanging Back

This exercise is highly effective because it stretches all the upper back muscles in one shot, including the lats, the trapezius, and the upper part of the erector spinae (you can stretch the lower part of the erector spinae by relaxing at the start position of the back extension exercise).

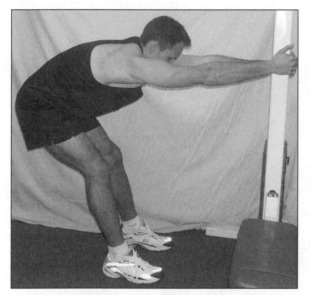

Extending your hips and butt, lean back with your entire body weight.

1. Hold on to a doorknob, a stretching bar, or the side of any heavy exercise machine at about waist height. Step back about 2–3 feet, and stand with your feet apart.

2. Drop your head down between your arms, and lean back as if you were going to try to pull the machine across the floor. Let your hips and butt extend behind you, using your entire body weight to stretch your back muscles. Hold this stretch for 15–30 seconds, stand back up to rest, and then repeat until you have completed a full minute.

Abdominal Reach

Beware of this exercise—after a vigorous workout, you may never want to get up from it! Try to do this stretch immediately after working your abs so the muscles aren't tight as you continue with other exercises.

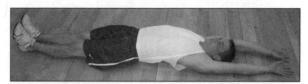

Stretch yourself from head to toe by reaching with your hands and pushing with your toes simultaneously.

1. Lie on your back on the floor. Keep your feet together and point your toes toward the ceiling. Reach out over your head with both arms, pointing your fingers away from you.

2. Try to make yourself as "long" as you can. Reach out with your hands, and push your feet away from you at the same time. If your back arches off the floor a little bit, that's okay—it means your abs are stretching. Hold for 15–30 seconds, relax, and repeat until you complete a full minute.

Glutes and Hips

Whenever you do isolated glute exercises or thigh exercises that require you to move at the hips (leg press, squat, and so on), be sure to stretch them afterward with this exercise.

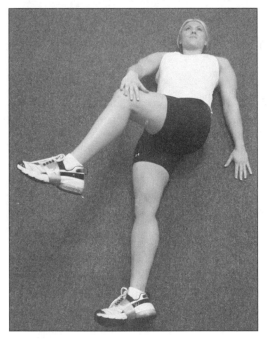

The more you pull on your knee, the more you'll feel this stretch.

1. Lie on your back on the floor, legs straight, with your arms beside you. Bend your left knee up and then reach up and grab it with your right hand. Your left arm and right leg stay on the floor.

2. Let your leg and foot relax, using your hand to support them. Pull your knee up and across your body to stretch your left hip and glutes. The more you pull your knee toward your shoulder, the more you will feel this stretch in your butt. Hold for 15–30 seconds and then switch and stretch the other side. Alternate legs until you have finished a full minute on each side.

Quadriceps Stance

When you begin doing thigh exercises, stretching the quadriceps afterward will become second nature because it feels so good to loosen up the muscles. With this exercise, you may not feel as much of the stretch "burn," but you will feel a relief of muscle tension.

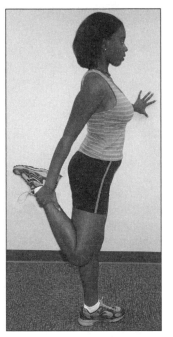

Hold the stretch for 15–30 seconds and then alternate legs.

1. Stand next to a wall or a machine that you can hold on to for balance. Bend one foot up behind you, and grasp your shin. Be sure you are holding on to your shin and not your foot—stretching and twisting the ankle can lead to injuries.

2. Keep your body as straight and tall as possible—don't lean forward during the stretch. Pull your foot up behind you as far as you can, letting your hip bend and your knee move backward. Hold the stretch for 15–30 seconds and then do the other leg. Alternate legs until you have a full minute on each side.

Hamstring Toe Touch

Every time you stretch your quadriceps, you must also stretch your hamstrings to keep your body in balance. Tight hamstrings lead to pulled hamstrings—and if you've ever had a pulled hamstring, you know it's no fun.

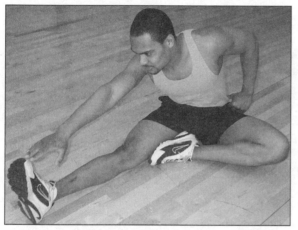

Don't worry if you can't touch your toes right away; that ability will come as you continue stretching.

1. Sit on the floor with your left leg straight and your right leg bent so your foot is against the inside of your knee.

2. Reach out with your left hand toward your toes. Let your body lean forward until you feel the stretch. It's okay if you can't touch your toes right now—that will come with practice. Hold the stretch for 15–30 seconds and then switch to the right leg. Alternate stretching each leg until you finish a full minute on each side.

Achilles Step

You should stretch your calves after performing any leg exercises or cardiovascular workout. Because your calves work all the time—anytime you take a step—they are almost always warmed up and ready to stretch.

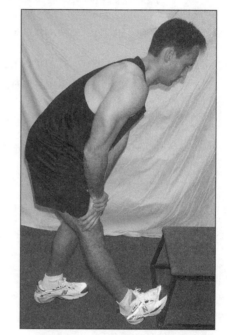

Lean your chest forward and your hips back to get a deep calf stretch.

1. Place your toe against a doorway opening, a wall, a pole, the edge of a step, or anything that won't move when you push against it. Keep that leg straight, and step back with the other leg to give yourself some stability and balance.

2. Place your hands on the knee of the leg you are going to stretch, lean your body forward, and let your hips move back and down a bit. You will feel this stretch from the back of your knee all the way down to your foot. Hold it for 15–30 seconds, switch legs, and repeat until you finish a minute on each side.

In This Chapter

◆ Why aerobic exercise is important for body sculpting

◆ Exactly how much aerobic exercise is right for your specific sculpting program

◆ Reaching your target heart rate

◆ Increasing time vs. increasing intensity

◆ The importance of cooling down

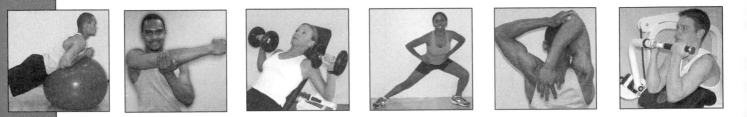

Chapter 8

Taking Exercise to Heart

In addition to proper nutrition and exercise, the third component of the body-sculpting program is moderate aerobic exercise. If the idea of aerobic exercise conjures up images of endless hours of sweating on a machine you detest, you've got the wrong idea. You can incorporate many activities into your body-sculpting routine that will be effective *and* enjoyable, and we'll discuss those alternatives in this chapter. But first, what exactly is aerobic exercise?

Aerobic exercise is all about working the most important muscle you have: your heart. In fact, your heart is your body's primary muscle. Without it, nothing else works. Aerobic exercise not only helps you build a strong heart, but it also helps you burn calories, which helps you lose fat and better reach your body-sculpting goals.

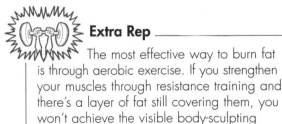

Extra Rep

The most effective way to burn fat is through aerobic exercise. If you strengthen your muscles through resistance training and there's a layer of fat still covering them, you won't achieve the visible body-sculpting results you're seeking.

Run, Bike, Swim, or Skate?

You can get the *aerobic* exercise you need in many ways, each of them beneficial. There is nothing magical about a treadmill or a stair-stepper and nothing life-changing about riding a bike; they are all just different ways of moving your body and working your heart, helping you burn calories.

Trainer Talk

Aerobic and cardiovascular exercise are one and the same: They both involve activity that raises your heart rate and burns more calories. This type of exercise is an important part of your body-sculpting regimen.

So what type of aerobic exercise should you do? Everything you can! Try every machine in the gym, and get outside and do different activities when the weather's nice. Go beyond what your body is used to, and find new ways of shedding extra pounds—while also having fun. Each type of aerobic exercise works different muscles in different ways. Some concentrate on the legs, some focus on the arms, and some put everything together to test your coordination as well. Here are some great body-sculpting options:

In the gym:

- Treadmills
- Stationary bikes
- Stair-steppers
- Ellipticals
- Cross-country ski machines
- Rowing machines
- Arm bikes
- Recumbent bikes
- Step-mills
- Aerobics classes

Outside:

- Walking or jogging
- Cycling
- Swimming
- Skating
- Rowing or kayaking
- Mountain biking
- Stair climbing

Start with the activities you feel comfortable with and already enjoy. Any activity can become boring or tedious (which means it will be harder to stick with for any length of time), so experiment with new gym equipment or outdoor activities to discover what you like to do. If you hate a certain machine, don't force yourself to use it. Choose an alternative, such as a group class or outdoor sport.

Another factor to consider when choosing your aerobic exercise is the number of calories it burns. Exercises that make you support your own body weight and move more of your muscles (working out on a treadmill, taking an aerobics class, skating) burn more calories than exercises done sitting down or using only some of your muscles (riding a stationary bike, using a stair-stepper or elliptical). If your goal is to lose extra fat, choose exercises that work as many of your muscles as possible (swimming, using a rowing machine, using a cross-country ski machine, jogging) so you can reach your goal faster. If you're maintaining your current fitness level, take advantage of less-strenuous exercises that don't burn as many calories.

Extra Rep

To choose your aerobic exercise, consider how many calories an exercise burns—plus what you enjoy doing. You won't stick with an exercise you don't like.

Time to Burn Some Fat

When you have decided what aerobic exercises you want to do, you need to devise a plan to get the appropriate amount of calorie-burning exercise for your body-sculpting goals. Most professional health and fitness organizations recommend between 20 and 60 minutes of cardiovascular (the fancy name for aerobic) exercise on most days of the week. How much time you spend on the aerobic part of your program is really determined by how much time you have, how intense you want to work, and what your goals are.

One of the most common excuses I hear from people who don't do any aerobic exercise is "I don't have enough time." But it's easier than you might think. If you are lucky enough to have a solid hour that you can devote to aerobic exercise, kudos to you. If you don't have an hour to work out all at once, divide your exercise into smaller parts. Doing two 30-minute sessions or four 15-minute sessions is just a beneficial as working out for a solid hour. It doesn't matter how many calories you burn all at once, as long as you burn them. A few minutes here and a few there add up to a lot of calories burned—just like eating a little here and eating a little there add up to a lot of calories stored.

The harder or more intense you work at your aerobic exercise, the less time it takes to burn the calories you need. This part is common

sense: If you work harder and move your muscles faster, you burn more calories. For example, you burn more calories jogging for a half-hour than walking for a half-hour. And every little bit helps. If you drove when you could have ridden your bike, or took the elevator instead of walked the stairs, it will take longer to reach your goals. Appendix E contains a list of popular exercises and the number of calories burned at different intensities.

The final factor in deciding how much time you spend on the aerobic part of your program is your individual goal. If you need to burn off some extra fat, here's the rule: To lose a pound of fat, you have to burn off 3,500 calories. A good and safe rate of weight loss is one pound a week. So if you want to lose a pound of fat each week, you need to burn 500 extra calories a day ($3,500 \div 7$ days). I don't recommend losing more than a pound of fat each week. Not only does it take a whole lot more aerobic exercise (more time, more stress on your body, less fun), but your body can adapt to slower weight loss easier than it can to rapid weight loss. Probably the most unsculpted look you can get is the saggy skin that results from losing too much weight too fast.

Extra Rep

To lose a pound of fat, you need to burn off 3,500 calories. To lose that pound in a week, choose an exercise that will burn 500 calories per day, and do it every day.

When you have reached your body-sculpting goals, or when you're comfortable maintaining your weight without losing more fat, you can adjust your exercise routines to burn only as many calories as you eat. This includes the calories burned from both resistance training and aerobic exercise. In reality, when you are at your target body-fat percentage, it takes very little aerobic exercise to maintain it (provided that you keep your calorie intake under control). Although the amount you need to burn may vary from day to day, try to do at least 30 minutes of aerobic activity to keep your heart in good shape.

Daily Dose of Cardio

Although almost all fitness professionals (myself included) recommend daily aerobic exercise, in real life, you may not have time for both aerobic and resistance training every day. Fortunately, doing resistance training also burns calories, although not as many as an aerobic workout. Try to do three to four aerobic workouts each week, plus resistance training, and you will make great progress toward a sculpted body. In fact, it's often a good idea to alternate your aerobic and resistance-training workouts on different days so your muscles have time to rest and recuperate between workouts. At the very minimum, two days of cardio a week will improve the strength of your heart, even if you're not burning off extra fat.

> **Extra Rep**
> By alternating your daily workouts between aerobic exercise and resistance training, you'll burn calories every day plus give your muscles time to recuperate.

In reality, very few people (usually only advanced athletes) can handle both aerobic workouts and resistance training on a daily basis. If you're a beginner, start with a minimum of two days of cardio a week and then add another day, and then another. By gradually adding more aerobic exercise by increasing the time or intensity, or changing the type of exercise, you'll burn more calories.

Harder or Faster

As I mentioned earlier in the chapter, the intensity of your aerobic exercise makes a difference in reaching your goals. Although it's true that you burn calories any time you move, certain levels of exercise will maximize your results without overly stressing or wearing down your body. You can determine the proper intensity for you in two ways:

♦ By using a certain percentage of your maximum heart rate

♦ By using a subjective measure called perceived exertion

Both methods can help you put your aerobic exercise plan into action and ensure that you are doing just the right amount of activity—not too much and not too little.

Counting Heart Beats

Because aerobic exercise is essentially exercise for your heart, it makes sense to base your intensity level on how hard your heart is working. Everybody's heart responds to exercise the same way: The harder the exercise is (pushing more weight, moving faster, using more muscles), the higher your heart rate will be. Designing your exercise program based upon heart rate is a tried-and-true method that fitness professionals have used for decades. This method is individualized for each person based upon age and resting heart rate. Using the following method, calculate a heart rate range that is right for you:

1. Determine your one-minute resting heart rate. It's best to sit down and rest for a few minutes to allow your heart rate to reach its lowest level. Measure your heart rate by using your index and middle fingers to find your pulse on either your wrist or your neck (see the following photos for clarification). Count your pulse for one minute.

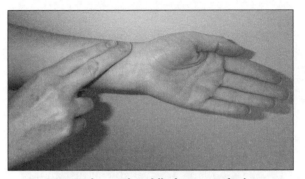

Use your index and middle fingers to find your pulse at your wrist. Your pulse point is in the groove just below your palm on the thumb side.

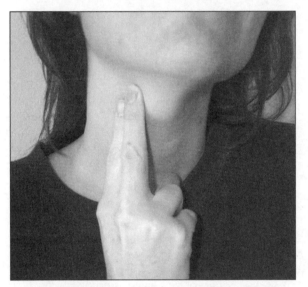

Use your index and middle fingers to find your pulse on the side of your neck. Your pulse point is in the groove just to either side of the center of your neck.

Extra Rep

For an ideal aerobic workout, aim to reach 60–80 percent of your maximum heart rate. At less than this, you won't burn enough calories; at more, you'll burn out too quickly.

2. Subtract your age from 220. This is an estimate of your maximum heart rate, the highest your heart rate can possibly go with intense exercise.

3. Subtract your one-minute resting heart rate from this number. The result is your heart rate reserve, the number of beats your heart rate can increase from resting to maximum effort.

4. Multiply this number by 0.6 and by 0.8. Here you are determining 60 percent and 80 percent of your heart rate reserve.

5. You now have two numbers. Add your one-minute resting heart rate to each of them. These numbers represent the low and high target heart rates for moderate aerobic exercise intensity—that is, your heart rate training zone.

Here is an example: Becki is 31 and has a resting heart rate of 72 beats per minute. She subtracts her age from 220 (220 − 31 = 189). Next, she subtracts her one-minute resting heart rate from 189 (189 − 72 = 117). She then multiplies 117 by 0.6 and 0.8 (117 × 0.6 = 70.2, 117 × 0.8 = 93.6). Finally, she adds her one-minute resting heart rate to each of these results (70.2 + 72 = 142.2, 93.6 + 72 = 165.6). Her moderate aerobic exercise heart rate training zone is approximately 142 to 166 beats per minute. This means Becki should exercise at an intensity that keeps her heart rate between 142 and 166 beats per minute.

This heart rate training zone is basically 60–80 percent of what your heart is capable of. Exercising below 60 percent still burns calories, but your heart won't see any benefit, and it will probably be so easy that you won't even know you're exercising. On the other hand, anything above 80 percent is too high. At this point, you start burning more carbohydrates instead of fat because you have to provide energy quickly to support the work you are doing, and fat is burned better at lower heart rates. Additionally, when you start exercising above 80 percent of your target heart rate, you won't be working out for long; you will become fatigued before you burn enough calories to make a difference.

So where in this heart rate training zone, ideally, should you aim for? There is obviously a difference between 60 and 80 percent. If you are starting your program after being relatively sedentary, stay in the 60–65 percent range until you become accustomed to your program and move up from there. If you've already been exercising a while, aim for the 70–75 percent range and go from there. No matter where you start, eventually your fitness level will improve and you'll need to increase your level of intensity.

When you get to the point that you finish a workout and don't really feel like you've worked that hard—you haven't really broken a sweat, or you feel like your muscles haven't gotten much of a workout—it's time to reach for a higher target heart rate. You should also intensify your workout if you aren't reaching your fat-loss goals and you feel that you can handle a tougher program. You'll burn more calories and get quicker results when you work at a higher heart rate. However, don't increase your exercise intensity before your body is ready. Jumping to the high end of the scale just to burn more calories isn't worth it if that exercise session wipes you out and makes you sore. Give your body a chance to get used to a certain level of intensity before ratcheting it up.

No Pain—Just Gain

Don't push your body too hard. Let your body adjust to one intensity before going faster, higher, or farther.

You can check your heart rate during your workout in two ways: You can manually check your pulse, or you can use a personal heart-rate monitor. Manually checking your pulse is a bit cumbersome if you are bouncing up and down or moving around too much. I prefer to use a personal heart-rate monitor, which is a great tool to have for your body-sculpting program. Heart-rate monitors have become very inexpensive ($25–$50) and are available at just about every sporting goods store or online (see Appendix B for some reliable sources). They will provide you with instant readings, and some can be programmed to alert you if your heart rate gets too low or too high.

How Hard Are You Working?

The second means of determining the appropriate intensity of an aerobic workout, as mentioned earlier in this chapter, is called a *rating of perceived exertion (RPE)*. Like a heart-rate training zone, an RPE, is individualized for each person. It is a subjective measure of how hard you feel you are working.

Trainer Talk

A **rating of perceived exertion,** or RPE, is another means of figuring out the appropriate intensity of your aerobic workout. Shoot for a rating of between 5–6—moderate to somewhat hard—during your workout.

An RPE has a holistic approach to reaching your target intensity, by combining all the feelings you have during an exercise into one number. Your current RPE is a measure of how hard you feel you are working, taking into account how hard you are breathing, how your muscles feel, how much you are sweating or how hot you are, and how much more you think you can take. RPE is measured on a scale of 1–10, with 1 being equivalent to absolutely no effort (lying down), and 10 being the highest level of exercise intensity you have ever felt. At an RPE of 10, you would feel that you are about to fall over; you can't go any farther or any longer—it's the absolute max. Here is how the scale ratings break down:

1: Nothing

2: Extremely light

3: Very light

4: Light

5: Moderate

6: Somewhat hard

7: Hard

8: Very hard

9: Very, very hard

10: Absolute maximum

A moderate level of aerobic exercise is equal to an RPE of 5–6 (moderate to somewhat hard). I add the "somewhat hard" rating to your training zone so you have a small range to work in. As you become more fit, you will increase the percent of your heart rate that you train at, but the RPE should stay the same. The exercise will always feel moderate to somewhat hard. If your workout ever becomes light, you know you need to bump it up a notch.

Remember that a rating of perceived exertion is different for everyone. What may be moderate for you might be very hard for someone else. This is a very individualized way of determining exercise intensity, but it's very useful when you switch forms of exercise. For instance, on a treadmill, you may feel moderate (RPE of 5) in your 70–75 percent heart rate zone, but when you go jogging outside, you may feel moderate in your 65–70 percent heart rate zone. Because

all exercises are not created equal, you will feel different and have a different comfortable training zone with each one. Using an RPE measurement is a good way to equate different exercises. If you are always between 5–6 on the RPE rating, then you know you are within your training zone and are making progress toward your sculpting goals.

Which Comes First: Time or Intensity?

As you are putting together the aerobic training part of your body-sculpting plan, you will come to a point at which you have to make a decision: "Should I increase the amount of time I train, or how hard I'm training in the time I have?"

The answer to this question depends on which of three possible scenarios fits you best:

◆ You aren't getting the full 60 minutes, but you cannot devote any more time to aerobic training.

◆ You are already at the 60-minute limit, so there isn't any more time to add.

◆ You're getting at least 30 minutes, but you probably have some room in your schedule to add more.

Intensity Before Time

If you are starting out with less than 60 minutes of total aerobic training time each day and you don't have any more room in your schedule to add more, concentrate on increasing the intensity of your workout before you try to lengthen it. This will allow you to burn more calories in the time you have already set aside. Consider adding more time only when you feel you're working as hard as you can.

If you are already at the 60-minute limit, consider increasing your intensity as well. Sure, you might be able to do more than 60 minutes of cardio at a time, and if you really want to, go ahead. But be warned that too much exercise can stress your muscles and joints to the point of injury, plus delay your body's recovery time.

So in these two scenarios, the rule is, intensity comes before time.

Time Before Intensity

If you aren't at the 60-minute limit yet, and you do have room in your schedule to add more time, do it. When you reach your personal time limit, you can increase the intensity. First, put in as much aerobic training time as you can.

Cooling It Down

The final part of your aerobic training workout should always include a good cool-down. Far too often, I see people get off the treadmill or bike, or come in from a jog, and go straight to flexibility training or, worse, go to the locker room and get dressed. Cooling down after having your heart rate up is very important.

Your heart is a pump; it pushes blood out. Your heart cannot suck blood back to it. When you exercise, your heart pumps a lot of blood to your muscles, and when your muscles contract, they squeeze the blood back to the heart. When you suddenly stop moving, all the blood that has been sent to your muscles stays there—very little of it gets back to the heart. This causes your heart rate to increase even more instead of slowing down, as it should after you exercise. This can lead to dizziness or lightheadedness and, in some cases, can even cause a heart attack.

Q&A

Is "cooling down" really so important?

It's important to lower your heart rate gradually rather than suddenly to avoid becoming dizzy or lightheaded, or even having a heart attack.

To cool down properly, spend time moving at a lower intensity until your heart rate returns to its resting level. If you've been jogging, cool down by walking. With cardio machines, reduce the intensity until your heart rate comes down. Walking is always a safe bet for a good cool-down.

The Least You Need to Know

◆ Choose an activity or machine that you enjoy, and you'll be more likely to stick with it.

◆ To lose a pound, you need to burn 3,500 calories. To lose a pound per week, add activity that will burn an additional 500 calories per day.

◆ For moderate aerobic activity, try to reach 60–80 percent of your maximum heart rate as you exercise.

◆ The longer and more intense your aerobic workout is, the more calories you'll burn.

◆ The rating of perceived exertion is a different way to measure the intensity of your workout and is beneficial for comparing different forms of exercise.

◆ Always cool down after an aerobic workout.

In This Part

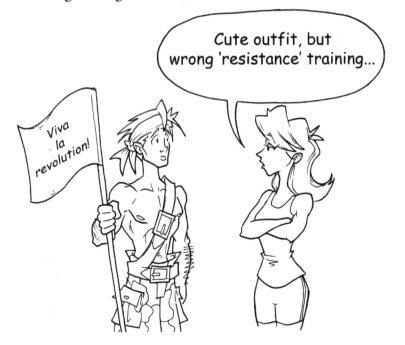

Part 4

Resistance Training: The "Tools" for Carving Your Physique

Just as a chisel makes a sculpture so much easier to shape, the tools for resistance training—weights, machines, tubing, and exercise balls—will help make your body that much easier to shape. Of course, an artist isn't born with the knowledge to perfect his craft; it takes work and training and the proper tools to make it happen. The following chapters simplify and demystify the craft of resistance training, with step-by-step instructions and photographs to lead you along the way to a stronger, healthier, and fantastic-looking body.

In This Chapter

- ◆ Avoiding injury during resistance training
- ◆ Maximizing repetitions and sets
- ◆ How much weight you should use with each exercise
- ◆ The importance of resting between sets and workouts
- ◆ Preventing boredom

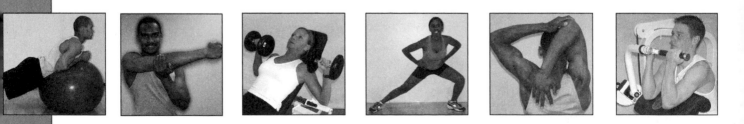

Chapter **9**

Resistance Rules

The absolute cornerstone of your body-sculpting program is *resistance training*. You've already learned how good nutrition will fuel your workouts, how stretching will release workout tension, and how aerobic exercise will burn excess fat. But focused, effective resistance training is the real key to unlocking your body-sculpting potential. This chapter outlines how to design a resistance-training program to meet your specific goals. The following chapters provide you with instructions and photographs detailing exactly how to do each exercise.

As with any other part of your body-sculpting program, understanding and proper planning are extremely important. You need to understand how the different components of a resistance-training program work together so you can achieve results without wasting time or effort.

Trainer Talk

Resistance training consists of weight-bearing exercises that directly build and strengthen your muscles, bringing you the body-sculpting results you seek.

Safety and Form

Getting hurt is the last thing you want when you are trying to improve your body. Injuries can occur at any time, in any place, and to anybody. Fortunately, the only time the body gets hurt is when you do something you shouldn't do, do something you weren't ready for, or do something the wrong way. If you follow the rules set out in this chapter and the instructions for each exercise, you should remain injury free. However, if you decide that there is an easier way of doing something (and there is always an easier way), you risk getting hurt. Easier is not always better—if body sculpting was that easy, everyone would look incredible.

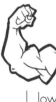

No Pain—Just Gain

It is extremely important to follow the safety precautions outlined in this chapter—and provided with each exercise in the following chapters—to prevent injury.

The first thing I always tell my clients as they learn a new exercise is "Nobody ever got hurt doing an exercise correctly and within their ability." This means that proper form is crucial and that you shouldn't attempt exercises that are too advanced for you. The human body is essentially lazy: It wants to get the job done as fast as possible with as little effort as possible. But as I said, fast and easy isn't always the best route.

Proper form means keeping moving body parts working correctly and keeping stationary body parts relaxed. With any exercise, there will be muscles that are active, muscles that are relaxed, and muscles that are helping to stabilize the body. For instance, during a biceps curl, the legs, abdominal muscles, and lower back muscles stabilize you to keep you standing; the arm muscles are working to move the weight; and the chest and back muscles are relaxed. If any of these muscles decide to do something else, the exercise will go wrong, and you risk injuring yourself.

Some of the exercises in this book are more advanced than others. To figure out whether a movement is too advanced for you without risking injury, try doing the exercise with just your body weight for resistance (no added weights). If you can't complete an exercise with just your body weight (body squats, for example), then you shouldn't try the same exercise with extra weight (such as barbell squats). You must be totally in control of your body and any added weight to perform an exercise safely.

No Pain—Just Gain

If done properly, no exercise should cause you injury. You risk getting hurt if you don't use proper form or if you do an advanced exercise you're not ready for.

Some of the exercises in the next chapters have a "Precautions" section that explains potential issues that may arise and what to do to prevent injury. Some exercises are potentially more dangerous than others, and some are almost foolproof. Regardless of how simple an exercise may seem, always pay close attention to each of the instructions, and follow them exactly to ensure a safe and productive workout.

Can You Spot Me?

One of the easiest and most vital precautions you can take with many resistance exercises is to use a *spotter*. A spotter is another person who can watch you do the exercise and be prepared to take control of the weight if you get into trouble. Use a spotter anytime you hold a weight over your head or chest that could fall and hit you. Most of these exercises call for lying on a bench or on the floor. Although it may be tempting to forgo using a spotter for the sake of convenience or a faster workout, this is an accident waiting to happen. It's too late to call for a spotter after the weight has hit you on the head or chest.

Trainer Talk

It's critical to use a **spotter** during certain exercises. This person will watch you do an exercise and take control of the weight if you suddenly can't.

Obey the Speed Limit

With very few exceptions, every exercise should be done at a speed you can control. To maintain control, you should be able to stop the movement at any time. For instance, if I walked up to you during an exercise and said "Stop," you should be able to stop immediately. If you have to slow the weight before you can stop it, you were not in control.

In addition to preventing injury, controlling the weight with slow, deliberate motion provides more effective sculpting results. The faster you move the weight, the more momentum you create. When you're using momentum as a force, you use your muscles less—or you need to use the wrong muscles to correct the movement. For instance, during a biceps curl, if you swing the weight and use momentum, at the

top of the movement, you have to activate your triceps to slow the weight before it hits your shoulder. This exercise is for the biceps, not the triceps. By using momentum to help lift the weight, you took some of the exercise away from the biceps and gave it to the triceps, thus reducing your body-sculpting benefits.

Extra Rep

A slow, controlled rate of lifting weight is not only safe, but it also provides more effective sculpting results. Avoid using momentum.

A safe and effective resistance training speed is always slow. To maintain the right speed, count two seconds up and two seconds down. During the bench press, for example, it should take you two seconds to lower the weight to your chest and two seconds to push it back up again.

Warming Up Your Engine

Before you embark on your daily resistance-training workout, it's important to get your body ready for the task at hand. Although your muscles are almost always ready to work, they aren't necessarily ready to work hard. That's why warming up each muscle group before you get into your workout is essential. Warming up provides more blood flow to the muscles, which equals more energy; helps loosen up the joints; and prepares your mind to send the proper signals to each muscle.

A proper warm-up can start with light aerobic exercise such as walking, jogging in place, or doing some simple calisthenics, such as jumping jacks. The idea is to get the body moving and get your heart rate up a little bit. After this initial warm-up, you should also warm up each specific muscle group you plan to work specifically.

Do this by performing a given exercise first without any added weight, just to get your muscles and joints moving with proper form. Then do a light set using only about one third of the weight you would normally use. These warm-ups shouldn't tire you out, and they won't decrease the results you get from your full workout. Instead, they should increase the benefit of each exercise. Unfortunately, these warm-up sets don't count toward your total exercise plan—they are a preventive addition.

Extra Rep

Be sure to warm up your whole body and your muscles individually before taking on your full resistance-training program.

Do your warm-up for each exercise in your program before you start your regular workout, or warm up each muscle group right before you do specific exercises—either way works fine. All in all, a total-body warm-up should take only about 10 minutes, but it's 10 minutes of preparation and injury prevention you should never skip. In the end, skipping this warm-up can result in less-effective body sculpting—after all, you can't sculpt your body if you become injured.

Setting Your Goals

Your resistance-training program is made up of several components:

- The exercises you choose
- The number of repetitions in each set
- The amount of weight you use with each exercise
- The number of sets
- How long you rest between sets

Adjusting any of these components affects the rest of them, so designing the right program for your goals is very important. Each of the following sections outlines how to design your workout according to your goals. As your body-sculpting program progresses, refer back to this chapter if you need to make adjustments to keep yourself on track.

So Many Exercises, So Little Time

As you flip through the next chapters, you will notice that for each body part, there are a number of exercises to choose from. So how many should you do, and which are most effective? Here's some perspective: Each muscle group in your body does one thing really well. For instance, the biceps' job is to bend the elbow. Because your elbow bends only one way, all the biceps exercises involve the same movement: bending the elbow. However, small differences even among these exercises can affect the overall outcome of your program. These differences may make one exercise more comfortable or enjoyable for you than another; this, in turn, determines how happy you are with your program and how likely you are to stick with it (it doesn't make sense to do exercises you don't enjoy). So choosing the correct exercises for you is really just a matter of trial and error. There are no best or worst exercises; they are all just a little different. You may dislike my favorite exercise, or it may not bring you the same results. Over time, you will determine which exercises are providing you with results and which ones you feel comfortable doing. You can then modify your program to reflect these preferences.

Extra Rep

Choose exercises that you like and that provide results over time. Don't be afraid to modify your program if it's not working for you.

So now that you've chosen your preferred exercises, how many of them do you need to do for each muscle group? In a perfect world, only one. However, our bodies aren't perfect, and there isn't an exercise yet that works every fiber in a muscle at its highest level. For this reason, it may take two, three, or even four exercises per muscle group to get the results you're seeking. There's no magic number, and even science hasn't determined the optimum number of exercises needed to maximize each muscle group. Instead, your goals and how much time you have to work out should determine how many exercises you can do for each muscle group. If it takes you 30 minutes to complete one exercise for each muscle group, and if 30 minutes is all you have, then choose the one exercise you like best.

On the other hand, there is a point at which you won't achieve better results by adding more exercises. Each exercise you do decreases a muscle's ability to do other exercises because it gets tired. You can't work a muscle forever, or even for more than a few exercises, before it starts to fatigue. You'll get diminishing benefits as you move on to each new exercise for the same muscle. If you are tired after doing one exercise but still have time for another one, you probably won't do very well on the second one because the muscle is already worn out. Overdoing it can result in injury or severe soreness that will prevent you from working out anytime soon, which won't help you reach your goals. So if your form is compromised because your muscles are tired, it's time to stop.

In the end, pick two or three of your favorite exercises for each muscle group. If you have time, do more than one exercise per muscle. Remember, though, that you have only so much energy available for that workout, and it has to be spread out over all the muscle groups. Don't become so tired working one muscle group that you can't finish your workout. You

can also vary the number of exercises you do for each muscle group, such as concentrating more on the upper body or the lower body.

Repetitions for Success

At the gym, you'll hear a lot about *repetitions*, or reps. A repetition counts as each time you complete a full range of movement for a particular exercise. Unfortunately, you won't get results doing one repetition per machine. Instead, your muscles require multiple repetitions for proper sculpting stimulation. But there is a limit to the number of repetitions you should do, and this number should ultimately reflect your goals. Here's how it breaks down:

◆ If your goal is to strengthen and sculpt your muscles, complete four to six repetitions per set.

◆ If your goal is to increase the size of your muscles for even greater sculpting, complete 7–12 repetitions per set.

◆ If your goal is to increase your muscle's endurance and definition, but not get a lot stronger or bigger, complete 13–15 repetitions per set.

Trainer Talk

A **repetition** reflects each time you complete a full resistance-training movement. For example, one ab crunch repetition consists of you crunching up and then lowering your body back to its starting position.

The number of repetitions you do per set (we'll talk about sets in a moment) ultimately determines how your program will turn out. Body sculpting can mean several different things: stronger and more sculpted, bigger and more sculpted, or sculpted with a lot of endurance.

The neat thing about a body-sculpting program is that you can choose different goals for each muscle group simply by changing the number of repetitions you do. If you feel that your arms and shoulders are strong and big enough but need more sculpting, you should use sets of 13–15 repetitions for those muscles. At the same time, you may want your legs to be a little bigger and more sculpted; in that case, you should do 7–12 repetitions for your leg exercises. It's totally up to you how you change and sculpt your body; just manipulate your reps to reflect your goals.

Add Some Weight

When you determine the number of repetitions you'd like to do, you can figure out how much weight to use. A basic rule of body sculpting is that weight and repetitions are inversely related. This is actually quite logical: The heavier the weight is, the fewer times you will be able to lift it. On the other hand, if a weight is really light, you can do many more repetitions. So the amount of weight you use depends on the number of repetitions you've chosen, which was based on your goals. (See why goals are so important?)

But how do you know how much weight to use the first time around? This actually takes some trial and error, plus a bit of record-keeping (keep those exercise logs handy). Initially, you should always use the lightest weight available. It's better to start light and increase the weight than to start too heavy and get hurt before you even get started.

Use this rule of thumb: If you are able to complete all the repetitions for a particular machine or exercise, you need to use more weight in your next workout. Far too often I see people using the same weight over and over, never trying to do more. But this practice only maintains your current shape; it does not improve it. When you are capable of completing a

set with a given weight, you need to increase the weight for further improvement. Your body is already capable of doing the work, so there is no stimulus to change. You have to overload your muscles in a progressive manner to keep seeing improvement.

A common thought among new clients is that if they lift heavier weights, they will get bigger muscles faster. They quickly learn that this is true only if their program is designed to increase muscle size, which happens only with sets of 7–12 repetitions. As long as you can lift the amount of weight you've chosen for the proper number of repetitions, you'll achieve your goals.

Finally, remember the old candy-bar jingle "Some days you feel like a nut; some days you don't"? I have always liked that saying because it sums up an interesting situation that will probably happen to you at some point: Some days you feel on top of the world. Your muscles are strong, you're in a good mood, the workout is going great, and you easily complete all your repetitions. You think it's time to move up the weight. So during the next workout, you increase the weight, and bam! You find that you are really having trouble—it's way too heavy, and you don't feel nearly as strong as during the last workout.

The truth is, some days everything just comes together and you have great workouts (some days you feel like a nut). Other days, you struggle just to get through it (some days you don't). The causes are varied: Maybe your mind is on job or family responsibilities, maybe you didn't get enough sleep, or maybe you didn't eat as well that day. Whatever the reason is, you aren't feeling as strong. Because of this, I recommend the two-workout rule before increasing your weight: If you complete all your repetitions during two consecutive workouts, increase the weight on the third. This way, you won't move up your weight prematurely.

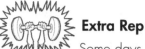

Extra Rep

Some days you'll just feel stronger and more energized than others, due to any number of factors. It could be a fluke, so before increasing your weight, be sure you can complete all your reps for at least two consecutive workouts.

Setting Up for More

A lot of controversy over the years has centered on how many *sets* you need to do for body-sculpting results. First, a set is defined as a full sequence of repetitions. For example, if you're looking to make your biceps bigger, one set includes 7–12 repetitions of a biceps curl. Most of the exercise routines you see in magazines and on TV recommend only one set, whereas most of the professional literature and research says that multiple sets are more effective. If you are new to exercise, one set will probably be enough to stimulate your muscles to improve—for a little while. After you have gotten into the groove of working out regularly, you'll need to complete two to three sets per exercise.

Trainer Talk

A **set** is a full sequence of repetitions. Doing one to three sets per exercise is the standard recommendation for body sculpting.

Increasing the number of sets is another way of creating a more challenging workout over time. Start with one set per exercise. When you've gotten to the point that you don't get results, try two sets per exercise. You can eventually move up to three sets, if you have the time. The benefits of the program will increase when you move from one set to two, and again when you move from two sets to three. Beyond that (four sets or more), though, the benefits are pretty much infinitesimal.

Again, you don't have to follow the exact same plan for all muscle groups. If you are happy with some muscles, doing one set per exercise will maintain those muscles' strength and form. For muscles that require more sculpting, use multiple sets per exercise until you are satisfied with the results.

Taking a Break

The final component of your resistance-training program is rest. Muscles can't be worked continuously; they require time to recuperate between sets and between workouts. Your goals, as well as your chosen number of repetitions, should determine just how much rest you take between sets. Here's how it works:

◆ When you are training for increased strength (doing between four and six repetitions), take two to five minutes of rest between each set. This is due to the heavier weights you're using.

◆ If your goal is increased muscle size (completing 7–12 repetitions), take only 30–90 seconds between sets. This maintains good blood flow to the muscles.

◆ When training for muscular endurance and definition, rest for 30 seconds or less. By its nature, endurance training means that you don't get to rest much, which can make for a really intense workout.

So how much rest should you get between workouts? The basic rule is 48 hours of rest between sessions, or resistance training done every other day. So if you work your biceps on Monday morning, you should wait until Wednesday morning to work them again. Training the same muscle any sooner cuts down on the time that muscle had to recover from the last workout, which can end up decreasing your long-term results.

Conversely, taking more than 72 hours (3 days) of rest is too much. When you work out, your body recognizes the additional stress and compensates by getting stronger and ready for the next workout. After 72 hours, if it doesn't experience similar stress, it thinks, "I don't have to be any stronger. That last workout was a fluke, so I'll go back to the way I was." As I said before, our bodies are lazy. To maintain and improve the results you have built, you should never go more than two days without working out. That means that if you exercise on Tuesday evening, you need to work out again by Friday evening. If you wait longer than that, your muscles will begin to lose some of the improvements from your last workout.

 Extra Rep

For best body-sculpting results, never go more than 72 hours between resistance-training sessions. Your body will begin to lose improvements if you don't consistently work these same muscles.

Using these rules, you actually have several options for planning your resistance-training workout. If you are going to do a full-body workout each session (exercises for all your muscle groups), here are some options using the every-other-day rule:

- Work out on Monday, Wednesday, and Friday; rest on Tuesday, Thursday, and weekends.

- Work out on Tuesday, Thursday, and either Saturday or Sunday; rest on Monday, Wednesday, Friday, and the other weekend day.

If you are going to divide your workout into two days (half your muscle groups on one day, and half the next), you can work out every day, alternating muscle groups, for instance:

- Monday, Wednesday, Friday: chest, triceps, shoulders, abs
- Tuesday, Thursday, Saturday: legs, biceps, back
- Sunday: rest

Of course, this rule is for resistance training only; you'll still need to add moderate aerobic exercise at least three days a week for optimal results.

Moving Forward

Progression is one of the key elements of a successful body-sculpting program. Without progression, you will maintain what you have but never improve. And what's the point of working out if you aren't going to make improvements? I actually know people who have been doing the same exact workout for years. They are perfectly happy with the time it takes them, the weight they lift isn't difficult, and they have a routine that they know by heart. The problem is, they also complain about not looking any better, and they don't understand how they can work out religiously but not make improvements. If you don't want to become one of these people (and I suspect that because you are reading this book, you don't), you must make regular progression in your workouts.

 Trainer Talk

Progression refers to consistently intensifying your workout so it remains a challenge, to bring continual improvements.

The key to progression first lies in your will to always do the best you can on every set, for every exercise, and during every workout. You can modify your progression first by increasing repetitions.

If you're working in a range of 7–12 repetitions per set, progress by striving for the maximum per set—12, not 10 or 7. When you can do this maximum number for two consecutive workouts, increase the weight. More weight may decrease your ability to do the maximum repetitions, so keep working until you are back to the maximum, ready to increase the weight again. This form of progression is easy to learn and remember because it resembles a circle (see the following figure).

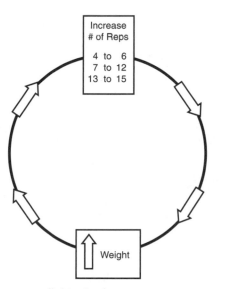

I call this circular progression.

Over time, as you become more sculpted, it will take longer to reach the top of the repetition range, and you won't increase the weight very often. That's fine, as long as you are always pushing yourself to do as many repetitions as you can in each set. If you do this and keep good track of it in your exercise log, you will always stimulate your muscles to improve. Using the two-workout rule explained earlier, along with circular progression, you should never hit a plateau, and you'll always be moving toward a more sculpted body.

No Boredom Allowed

I never fail to be both amazed and distressed when I hear that someone has quit working out because he or she became bored with it. There is absolutely no reason for this. If you flip through the next 10 chapters, you will see enough exercises to keep you busy for the rest of your life. Certainly, anyone can get bored doing the same exercises day in and day out, month after month, year after year, which is why you shouldn't do the same exercises all the time. Variety is the spice of life and also the key to keeping your workouts interesting.

 Extra Rep

It's natural to get bored if you do the same workout day in and day out. Be sure to add some variety to keep both your mind and your body stimulated for the long run.

Not only does your mind become dulled when you don't change your program, but your body gets accustomed and bored with your workout as well. As with any new activity, your body and mind work together to find the easiest way from point A to point B. In the case of your workout, you body learns to conserve energy, and you become extremely efficient in your movements. Although it's good to become efficient, you want to burn energy, not conserve it. You can ensure that you're burning the maximum amount of energy in two ways: Change the order of the exercises, or change the exercises themselves.

For instance, if you work out in the gym, avoid moving through your exercises in a specific order day after day. I like to call this the order of inorder. Move from exercise to exercise in random patterns, never doing the same thing twice. If you have 10 exercises in your workout, there are hundreds of ways of ordering them. This pattern can actually be more convenient in the gym, where you can never predict what machine or weights will be available from one moment to the next.

If you exercise at home or somewhere other than a gym, do the same thing: Scramble your exercises as much as you can. Make your workout random by writing all the exercises on pieces of paper and drawing them out of a hat. The first one out is your first exercise, the second is second, and so on.

To prevent mind and muscle boredom, you can also change the exercises in your program. As you become more proficient, change your exercises to more advanced lifts. I always suggest a total program change at least every three months. Learn a few new exercises, bring back some old ones, and add a new twist to those you want to keep. There are enough exercises in this book to change your program over and over, and this is just a sample of all the possible exercises available to you. Appendix E contains a few sample progressions of how you can change your workout over time.

The Least You Need to Know

- ◆ By using proper form at all times, you can avoid injury.
- ◆ Be sure to use a spotter when lifting weight over your head or chest.
- ◆ By controlling the weight with slow, deliberate motions, you will prevent injury and maximize your results.
- ◆ Choose the number of repetitions you do based on your specific body-sculpting goals.
- ◆ Weight should be determined through trial and error; too little, and you won't stimulate the muscles, and too much, and you risk injury or ineffective workouts.
- ◆ Be sure to rest between sets and between workouts. Forty-eight hours between each resistance-training session is ideal.

In This Chapter

◆ Where's your six-pack?

◆ Building strength at the center of your body

◆ Lying down and breathing for good form

◆ Bending and twisting to stronger abdominal muscles

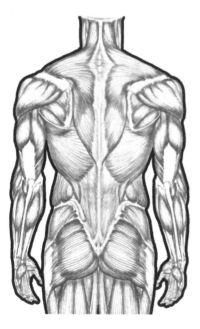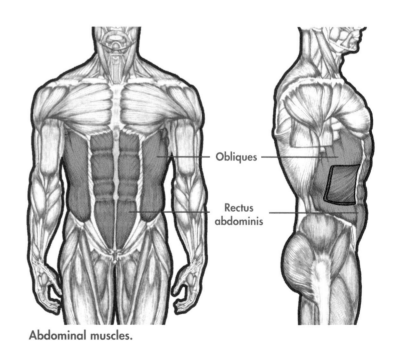

Obliques

Rectus
abdominis

Abdominal muscles.

Chapter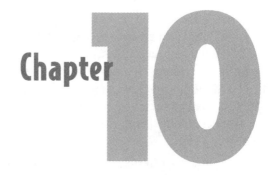

Absolute Abs

I usually can't go a single day without someone coming up to me, rubbing his or her belly, and asking, "How do I get these muscles in better shape?" My reply usually involves something like, "Put down that jelly donut and start doing crunches." Unfortunately, the jelly donut usually gets eaten instead of thrown away.

Lately, it seems you can't get away from people showing off their abs, whether you're picking up a fitness magazine, watching TV, or just walking through the mall. I would, too, if I had 2 percent body fat and the holy grail of muscle definition—the six-pack abs. The most inspiring thing I can tell you about your abdominal muscles is that you already have six-pack abs. Everyone does. The problem is that most of us have some fat lying on top of those muscles and getting in the way when we look in the mirror. All abdominal muscles are laid out in a "six-pack" arrangement, so we all have them. Getting to actually see them is another story and involves a combination of following a good nutrition plan, losing the excess body fat stored on the belly, and defining the abdominals through proper body-sculpting exercises.

The Most Important Muscle!

A couple years ago, fitness professionals shifted their thinking about what they considered the most important muscle group to train. The old idea was that whatever muscle was needed to move a particular weight was the most important. Athletes trained according to which muscles were needed to run, throw, jump, or shoot baskets.

The current thinking, however, is that the abdominals are always the most important muscle group, no matter what your goals are. Why? Because the abdominals make up the center of your body, also known as your core. Everything you do starts with your core and is supported by your abdominals. There isn't an exercise in this book that isn't affected by your abdominals, so be sure your body business plan includes a hefty dose of these targeting exercises.

Lie Down and Breathe

One of the greatest things about working your abdominal muscles is that you don't need any equipment or weights; you need just a floor. Of course, that also means you have no excuse for skipping this exercise. If you don't like to get on the floor, or if you have difficulty getting up and down off the floor, you can perform any of these exercises lying in your bed, on the couch, or on an exercise bench.

One of the most important things to remember when doing any type of abdominal exercise is to breathe out when you lift up. The abdominal muscles help you exhale. Every time you breathe out, cough, or sneeze, your abdominals contract. You can use this to your advantage by breathing out while you contract the muscles to squeeze every last bit of exercise out of them that you can. If you hold your breath, you are cheating yourself out of extra benefits, and it will take longer to reach your goals. Pretend there is a candle on a shelf above you while working your abs. Each time you contract the abdominals, try to blow out that candle with a quick, forceful breath. Try this technique with each of these exercises, and you will definitely feel the difference.

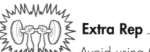 **Extra Rep**

Avoid using the body's momentum when performing abdominal exercises. Focus on working the abs during every crunch.

A Daily Dose?

Two schools of thought exist on how often and how much you should work your abdominal muscles. School number 1 dictates that the abdominal muscles are mainly an endurance muscle because they work every time you breathe; as such, you can exercise them every day. School number 2 theorizes that the abdominal muscles should be treated like every other muscle group and given a day of rest in between workouts. To date, there really isn't a clear answer as to which philosophy is correct. Athletes and nonathletes have achieved great results with both methods. The main factor in deciding whether you should work your abs every day is whether your body business plan includes time to work your abs every day. At the very least, you should perform abdominal training every other day.

No Pain—Just Gain

Unfortunately, abdominal exercises alone will not achieve muscle tone that you can see in a mirror. Sculpting the waistline also involves burning off abdominal fat through cardiovascular exercise, combined with good nutrition.

Where Are Your Abs?

The figure at the beginning of this chapter shows that your abdominal muscle is actually three separate muscles. The rectus abdominis is the one that has the six-pack look to it. It runs from the bottom of your ribs to the top of your pelvis. A common misconception is that you have "upper" and "lower" abdominals. The truth is that it's one muscle, and any abdominal exercise works both the "upper" and "lower" parts of the muscle equally. On some exercises, you may feel more of a burn on the top or bottom of the muscle, but that just indicates where the muscle is under the most strain—it doesn't mean that the rest of the muscle is relaxing.

The other two muscles that make up your core are the oblique abdominal muscles that run along the sides of your body, just under your ribs. The obliques help when you bend over forward, and they really work when you twist or turn from side to side.

Basic Crunch

The crunch is the mainstay of all abdominal exercises. The crunch involves all the muscles in your core, including your rectus abdominis (the six-pack part) and your oblique abdominals (right under the "love handles"). The crunch is really the first part of the old sit-up, but it doesn't require a partner or a heavy object to anchor your feet. Of all the exercises you will ever do, the crunch probably involves the least amount of actual movement, but it's a small movement that packs a punch.

Preparation

1. Lie down on your back on a carpeted surface, or use an exercise mat.
2. Bend your knees and keep your feet flat on the floor. Your heels should be placed no more than a foot away from your butt.
3. Cross your arms over your chest. If you want to put your hands on the side of your head, that's okay as well. However, do not lock your hands together under your head or support your head with your hands.

Movement

4. Take a deep breath and, as you blow it out, roll your head and shoulders off the ground toward your knees. You have to go up only about 30°, or to the point where you start to feel your shoulder blades leave the ground. Your lower back should stay on the floor.
5. Slowly lower yourself back to the ground, take a new breath, and repeat the process.

Precautions

◆ If your neck muscles get tired and you feel like your head is getting heavy, rest for a moment. You shouldn't lock your hands behind your head or support your head in any way because the crunch is also a good way to strengthen the neck muscles. In the beginning, those neck muscles may be weak and may get tired before your abdominals do, so let them rest and then begin exercising after a few breaths. And don't worry—you won't develop a big football player–like neck. You'll just make the muscles already there a bit stronger.

◆ Avoid jerking movements in an attempt to get in a couple more reps. The abdominal muscles like to work in smooth motions, and jerking them can cause the back muscles to contract and spasm.

Variations

A time will come when you can do crunches until you get totally bored. As the abdominal muscles get stronger, you will need to find other ways to stimulate them to work harder.

Add extra weight to your lift by holding a dumbbell, a medicine ball, or ankle weights under your chin. Be careful not to strain your neck muscles with too much weight. Five to fifteen pounds is plenty.

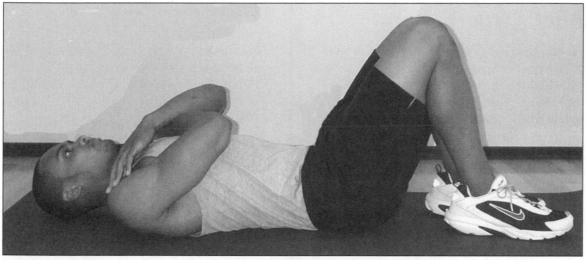

Starting/ending position.

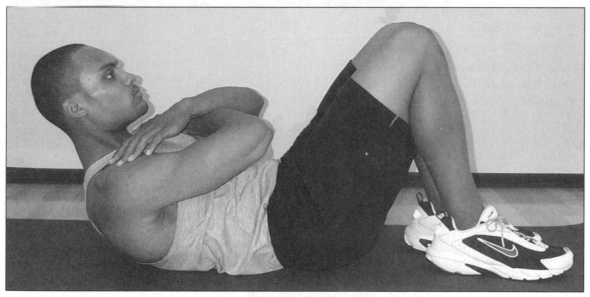

Midpoint position.

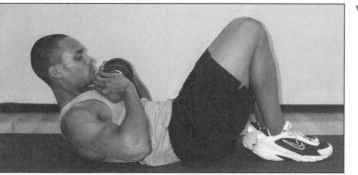

Variation.

Oblique Crunch

This exercise gets you ready to do the twist. The obliques are the abdominal muscles that work when you turn around to look behind you. This exercise gives the sides of your body a sculpted look. For you guys, this creates the taper from your shoulders down to your hips. For the gals, oblique crunches help better define an hourglass shape.

Preparation

1. Lie down on your back on a carpeted surface, or use an exercise mat.

2. Bend your knees and keep your feet flat on the floor. Your heels should be placed no more than a foot away from your butt.

3. Place one hand on the floor beside you and the other hand across your chest so your fingers touch the opposite shoulder.

Movement

4. Twist as you roll up so that the arm and shoulder that are lying on the floor stay on the floor, while the other side rolls up until that shoulder blade is off the floor. Remember to breathe out as you lift. It's almost like you are trying to roll over, but your hips and one shoulder are glued to the floor.

5. Lower yourself back to the floor, and begin again.

6. This exercise works only one side of your body at a time. After you've done a set on one side, switch your hands and go the other way.

Precautions

If you suffer from low back pain, or your doctor has told you that you shouldn't twist your body, skip this exercise. When you do oblique crunches, you are also moving your lower vertebrae (the lumbar section) in a twisting fashion. If you experience any pain during this exercise, stop and consult your doctor.

Variations

When you can do oblique crunches without much effort, add some weight to the shoulder being lifted. Hold a dumbbell, medicine ball, or ankle weight on that shoulder as you crunch. Five to fifteen pounds is plenty.

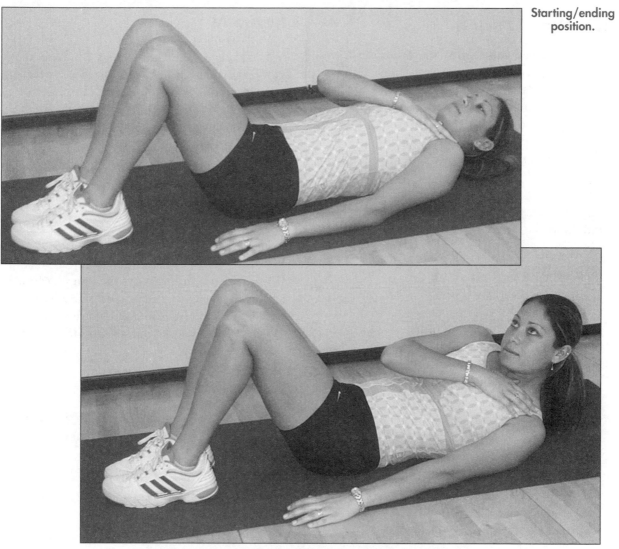

Starting/ending
position.

Midpoint position.

Variation.

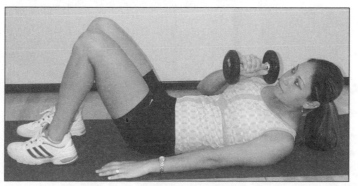

Balance Crunch

If we take away your ability to anchor the crunch with your feet, we create a new exercise called the balance crunch. This exercise is a bit more demanding because you will feel the abdominals working to keep you from rolling over as you crunch. You must crunch and maintain balance at the same time. If you do this exercise incorrectly, you will find yourself lying on your side, which doesn't do much for the abs. It may take some practice, but you'll find it a rewarding challenge.

Preparation

1. Lie down on your back on a carpeted surface, or use an exercise mat.
2. Bend your knees and lift your legs so it looks like you're sitting in a chair that fell over. Cross your arms over your chest.

Movement

3. Take a deep breath and, as you blow it out, roll your head and shoulders off the ground toward your knees. You have to go up only about 30°, or to the point that you start to feel your shoulder blades leave the ground. Your lower back should stay on the floor.
4. Slowly lower yourself back to the ground, take a new breath, and repeat the process.

Precautions

If you feel any strain or tiredness in your lower back while doing these crunches, put your feet back down and rest. You shouldn't feel anything in your back because your abs are doing all the work.

Variations

This exercise can be more difficult if you put your feet straight up instead of bending your knees. By making it even harder to balance, you'll challenge your abs more.

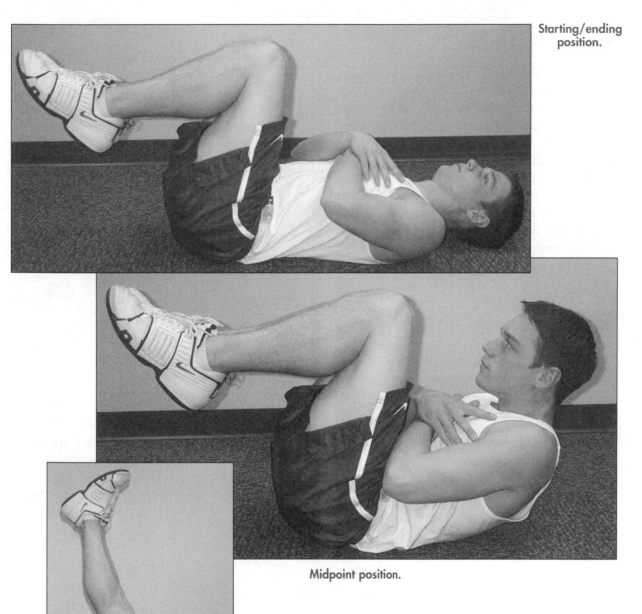

Starting/ending position.

Midpoint position.

Variation.

Reverse Crunch

The lower part of your abdominal muscles is not stressed very much during basic crunches or oblique crunches because the upper part is straining against the weight of your upper body while the lower part is anchoring the exercise. So to work the lower part a bit harder, you need to do crunches in reverse—that is, use butt raises. These are the muscles directly under that belly pooch many of us complain of, and they are the muscles you will see when you get rid of that extra layer of fat. When you do these correctly, you should feel the "burn" in your lower abs.

Preparation

1. Lie down on your back on a carpeted surface, or use an exercise mat.
2. Put your hands behind your head, and rest your elbows on the floor. You aren't going to be raising up your head, so having your hands behind your head is okay this time.
3. Bend your knees and lift your legs so it looks like you're sitting in a chair that fell over.

Movement

4. Slowly roll your hips up and off the floor while you breathe out. When done correctly, you'll feel like you're rolling into the fetal position. I like to think about bringing my knees toward my chin to keep me focused on the movement.
5. Stop rolling up when you feel your lower back start to lift. You don't want to go any farther than this. Roll up slowly so that momentum doesn't carry you too far. Although the movement is small, it's very beneficial.
6. Slowly lower your hips back to the floor, but keep your legs up and ready for the next repetition.

Precautions

It is extremely important that you do this exercise slowly. Do not use momentum to roll yourself up or in an attempt to do a few extra reps. When you are using your abdominal muscles, the back muscles should be resting. "Jerking" or moving too quickly can cause the back muscles to contract, which can end up causing injury.

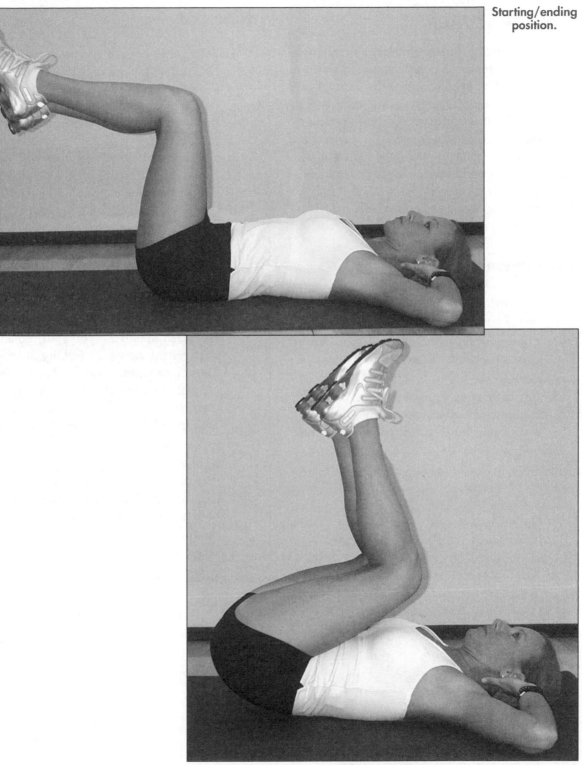

Starting/ending position.

Midpoint position.

Double Crunch

If you're looking for the ultimate ab challenge, look no further than the double crunch. Because you are combining elements of the basic crunch and the reverse crunch at the same time, this is probably the most difficult of the abdominal exercises. This is also a highly efficient exercise because you're working the entire abdominal muscle—upper and lower—with one exercise. When you do it correctly, you will feel the burn throughout the abs (and you'll probably be calling me names, too).

Preparation

1. Lie down on your back on a carpeted surface, or use an exercise mat.

2. Hold your legs straight up without lifting your hips off the floor. It's like you are trying to put your feet on the ceiling.

3. Put your arms straight up, too. During the movement, you are going to try to touch your toes, so aim your fingers now.

Movement

4. Take a deep breath and, as you blow it out, roll your shoulders up until the shoulder blades leave the floor, and roll your hips up until your butt is off the floor. Crunch from both ends at the same time, pushing your feet toward the ceiling and trying to touch your toes with your hands. The only thing left touching the floor is your lower and middle back.

5. Slowly unroll yourself back to the starting position.

Precautions

◆ Perform this exercise slowly, and take very deep breaths. If you get tired and start getting sloppy by jerking or trying to use momentum, stop and rest. Lack of control can cause the lower back to contract, which will cause you to work your back muscles instead of your abdominals.

◆ Don't worry if you can't reach your toes right away. You are pushing your feet farther up at the same time, so you really have to crunch the upper part of your body to reach. As your abs get stronger, the movement will become easier and you'll be able to crunch fully.

Starting/ending position.

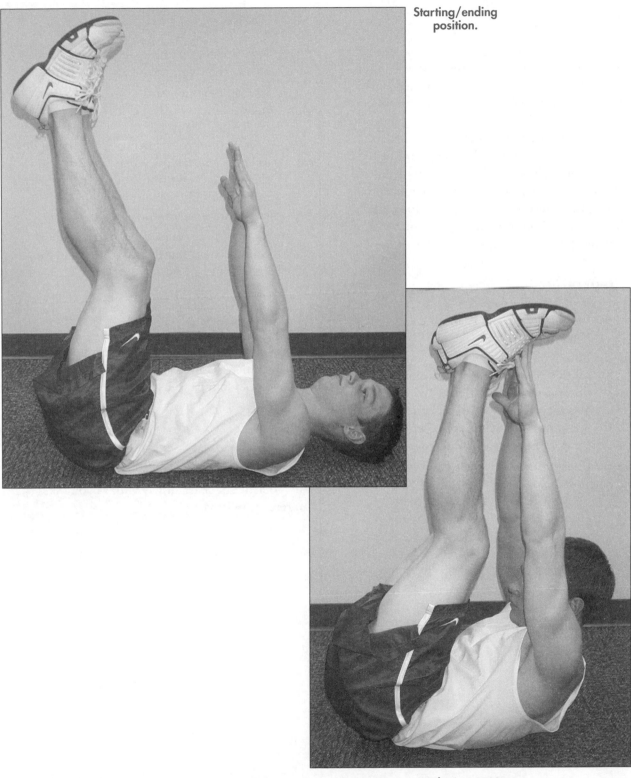

Midpoint position.

Rocky Abs

These abdominal exercises were inspired by Sylvester Stallone's character in *Rocky*. In the movie, Rocky did all kinds of unusual and challenging abdominal exercises that took serious strength. I don't recommend trying all his exercises (especially the crunches while hanging over the edge of a loft), but he performed a really effective oblique exercise that I call Rocky Abs. (*Note:* There is no guarantee that doing this exercise will make you look like Sylvester Stallone—or help you win a boxing championship.)

Preparation

1. Lie down on your back on a carpeted surface, or use an exercise mat.
2. Bend your knees and keep your feet flat on the floor. Your heels should be placed no more than a foot away from your butt. You may need to have someone hold your feet down, or anchor your feet under something heavy (such as your refrigerator).
3. Cross your hands over your chest.

Movement

4. Roll straight up until your shoulder blades are off the floor, just like a basic crunch.
5. Instead of going back down, twist your body as far to the left as you can go, kind of like you are trying to see what's on the floor behind you. Then twist to the right as far as you can go. Repeat twisting to the left and right until the abs really start to burn. While you are twisting, keep breathing in and out.
6. Slowly lower yourself back to the floor, take three or four deep breaths, and then do it again.

Precautions

If you feel your back muscles straining during or after this exercise, slow down your twists; use your abdominal muscles only to avoid injury.

Variations

You can intensify your Rocky Abs by speeding up your twists. Start slowly and, as you build intensity, twist faster.

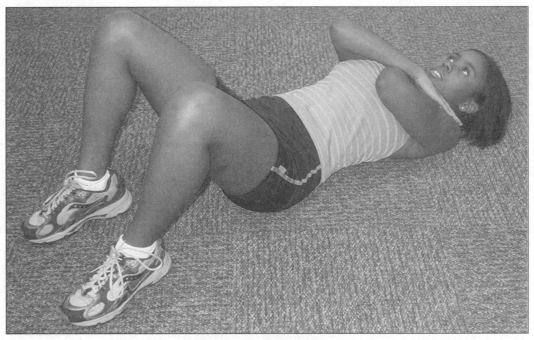

Starting/ending position.

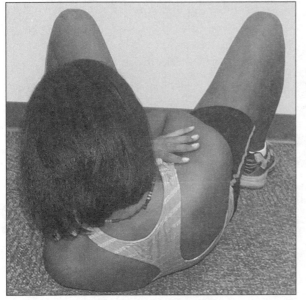

Midpoint position—left.

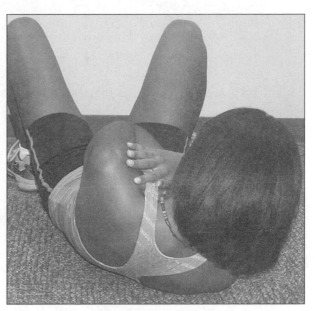

Midpoint position—right.

Abdominal Machines

The abdominal weight machine is probably the most used piece of equipment in any gym. As I said before, you can get a great workout from floor exercises, but the abdominal machines provide an additional means of resistance: more weight. There are two main variations of the abdominal machine: the kind with a padded bar across your chest, and the kind with padded elbow rests. Either type is fine and accomplishes the same thing: stronger abs. If you get tired or bored of doing floor crunches, or if you just don't like lying on the floor with a lot of people walking around, weight machines are a good option.

Preparation

1. Before you sit down, adjust the seat height to its optimum level. On each machine is a pivot point that is usually pointed out for you on the machine's instruction card. Adjust the seat so that your hips line up with this pivot point. This way, both you and the machine will bend at the same point at the same time.

2. Choose the weight you will use from the stack, making sure that the selector pin is inserted all the way.

3. If the machine has the padded bar across your chest, grab hold of the handles on the bar, or simply "hug" the bar to get your arms out of the way. If the machine has elbow pads, it will also have handles to hold on to. Place your elbows on the pads, and hold on to the handles in a comfortable position. See the following photos for an example.

Movement

4. Bend at the waist, and curl yourself into a ball (don't forget to exhale as you perform the movement). You really can't do the movement incorrectly on these machines because they have a set pattern of movement; all they require is for you to provide the muscle to do the moving.

Precautions

◆ If the machine has foot straps or a bar for you to anchor your feet, don't use them; they will cause you to use your hip flexor muscles instead of your abs and will weaken your workout. Place your feet flat on the floor or on the platform provided.

◆ Your abs are not designed to move large amounts of weight—just the weight of your upper body. That means that when you're using an ab machine with a large stack of weights, you'll always require the use of additional muscles. When performing the exercise, try to concentrate on using your abs as much as you can.

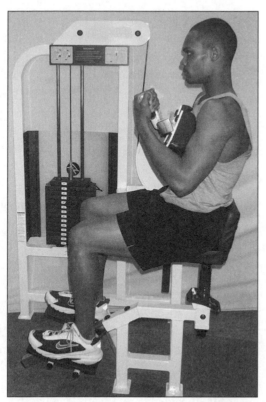

Starting/ending position—machine with padded chest bar.

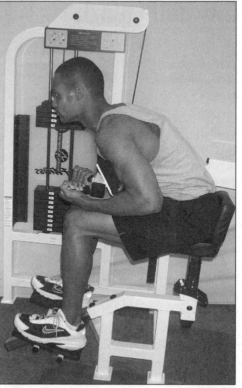

Midpoint position—machine with padded chest bar.

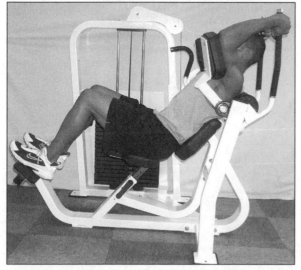

Starting/ending position—machine with elbow pads.

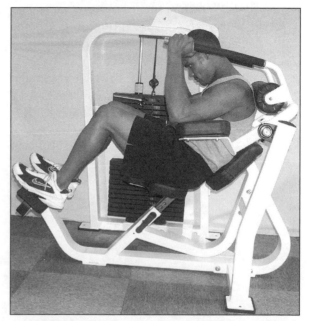

Midpoint position—machine with elbow pads.

Stability Ball Crunch

As I mentioned earlier in the chapter, no movement can be performed without the cooperation of the abdominals. Probably the hardest way to work your abs is on an unstable surface such as a stability ball. The ball forces all your core muscles to work together at the same time. It doesn't matter what size ball you have, as long as it is firm enough that you won't sink into it like a beanbag chair.

The ball crunch is essentially the same as the floor crunch, except that you are balancing on top of a ball. A benefit of the ball crunch is that you actually start the crunch in a position in which your abs are slightly stretched. This lets the muscles work over a longer period of time through a wider range of motion, which means you get more out of the exercise (that's more benefit, not more pain).

Preparation

1. Lie on the ball so that the top of the ball is in the middle of your back. Cross your hands over your chest.

2. Place your feet in a position in which you feel comfortable and balanced. A wide stance with your legs far from the ball will be more stable, and a narrow stance close to the ball will be unstable. The closer your feet are together—and to the ball—the harder you'll work your core.

Movement

3. Place your arms across your chest, take a deep breath, and breathe out as you roll up.

4. Stop when you feel your lower back start to come up off the ball. You can't use your shoulder blades as a measure of where to stop because they will be off the ball most of the time.

5. Slowly lower yourself back to the starting position, take a deep breath, and do some more.

Precautions

◆ If you find yourself sitting up with just your butt on the ball, you've gone too far.

◆ This is an advanced exercise, so if you seem to be rolling around on top of the ball, you need to spread your feet wider for more balance. Or go back to the basic floor crunch for a little longer to strengthen your abs.

◆ It's usually a good idea to do this exercise on a carpeted or padded floor, in case you slip off the ball.

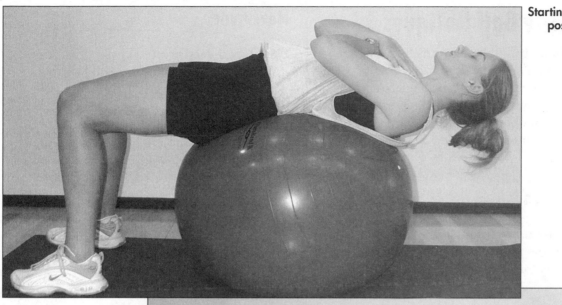

Starting/ending
position.

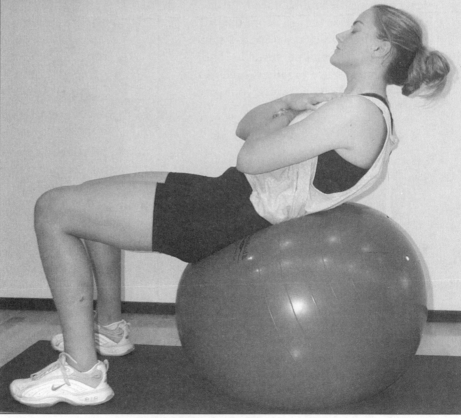

Midpoint position.

Stability Ball Obliques

The stability ball oblique works both sides of your obliques and challenges your ability to balance. Unlike the regular oblique crunch on the floor, with the stability ball, you alternate left and right oblique crunches. This gives one side a moment to rest while you crunch the other side.

Preparation

1. Lie on the ball so that the top of the ball is in the middle of your back. Cross your hands over your chest.

2. Place your feet in a position in which you feel comfortable and balanced. A wide stance with your legs far from the ball will be more stable, and a narrow stance close to the ball will be unstable. The closer your feet are together—and to the ball—the harder you'll work your core.

Movement

3. Take a deep breath. As you breathe out, lift your left shoulder up and twist your body to the right. Stop when you feel your lower back start to come up off the ball. You don't want to completely roll over.

4. Slowly return to the start position and take another breath.

5. Breathe out, lift your right shoulder up, and twist your body to the left. Stop when you feel your lower back start to come up off the ball. You don't want to completely roll over this way, either.

6. Repeat oblique crunches from side to side.

Precautions

◆ If you seem to be working your way off the ball, stop and reposition yourself. You need to keep the ball situated in the middle of your back between your shoulder blades.

◆ It's usually a good idea to do this exercise on a carpeted or padded floor, in case you slip off the ball.

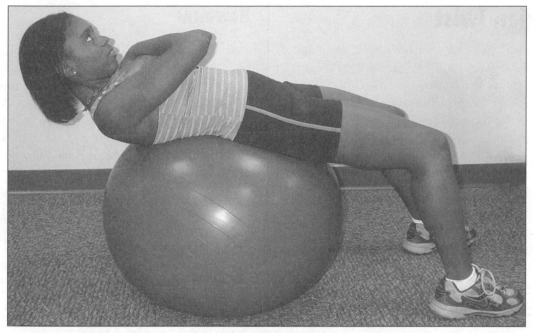

Starting/ending position.

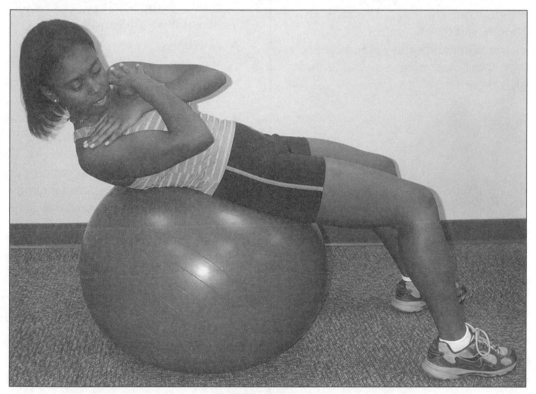

Midpoint position.

Russian Twist

A great way to work your obliques using a stability ball and resistance tubing is the Russian
twist. I believe this exercise got its name because
it mimics the famous Russian twist dance, but
nobody knows for sure.

Preparation

1. Sit on your stability ball (or a chair, if you
   don't have a ball handy). Place your feet a
   comfortable width apart—farther apart
   for more stability, closer together for less
   stability (but a more challenging movement).

2. Anchor your resistance tubing to a heavy
   machine or a doorknob.

3. Grasp the tubing with both hands just
   out to one side of your body a bit. The
   straighter your arms are, the more resistance you will feel. The band should have
   some tension in it at this point (there isn't
   any benefit in the movement if there isn't
   some tension).

Movement

4. Pretend you are swinging a baseball bat in
   slow motion. Breathe out and twist your
   entire upper body away from the tubing,
   as if you are going to turn around. At the
   same time, pull on the tubing, trying to
   stretch it across your body. As you twist,
   you will feel the band become more difficult to stretch.

5. Keep twisting until you are looking directly
   to your side. Then slowly return to the
   starting position, take a deep breath, and
   start over.

Precautions

- If your hips are rolling around on top of
  the ball, or if you don't feel comfortable
  sitting on the ball, use a chair until your
  obliques get a bit stronger.

- Anytime you use resistance tubing, be
  sure you have a good grip on it. It's just a
  big rubber band that will snap if you let
  go of it.

- If you suffer from low back pain, or if
  your doctor has told you that you shouldn't
  twist your body, skip this exercise. Russian
  twists also move your lower vertebrae (the
  lumbar section) in a twisting fashion. If
  you experience any pain during this exercise, stop and consult your doctor.

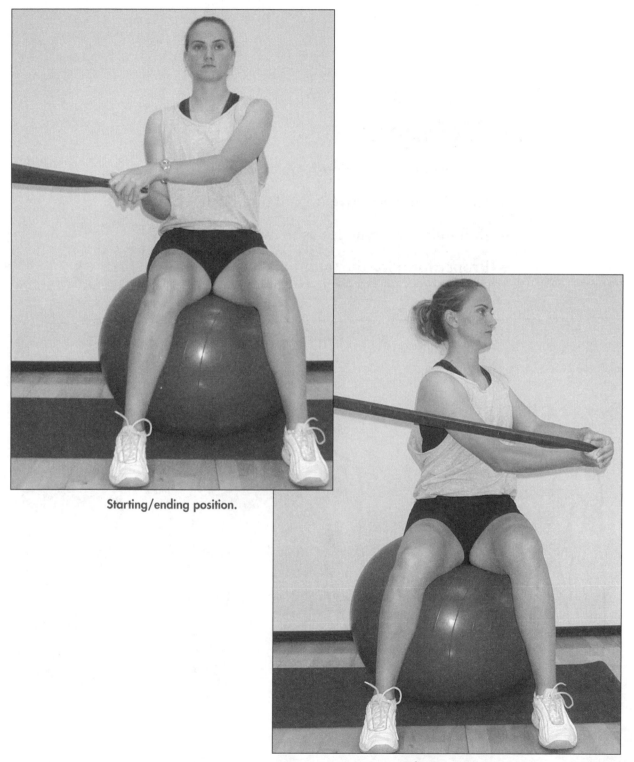

Starting/ending position.

Midpoint position.

In This Chapter

◆ Mastering the basic push-up

◆ Creative and effective uses of dumbbells

◆ Building chest muscles using weight machines

◆ Proper form for the traditional bench press

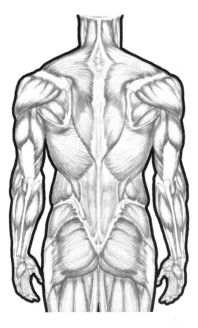

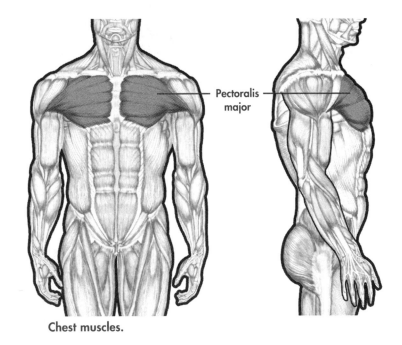

Pectoralis major

Chest muscles.

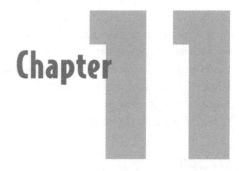

Chapter 11

Pecs to Be Proud Of

Here's a trivia question for you: What is the standard by which men judge other men? If you said the kind of car they drive or how big their tool collection is, you're wrong. In the gym, the standard you're measured by is "How much do you bench?"

Unfortunately, this standard provides bragging rights only until a stronger person enters the room. If you want to improve your score on this test of manliness, or if you simply want to give your chest a more sculpted look (my preference), this is the chapter for you.

Your chest muscles, formally known as your pectorals (and called pecs by the cool kids), are the main muscles that give football players the power to push each other around and give you the ability to do more practical things, such as push open doors and give hugs. For you gals, chest exercises are also important for defining your bust, highlighting your shoulder muscles, and, when a woman has had a mastectomy, regaining lost mobility and strength. Here's a great idea: Put those pecs to use right now and give yourself a hug for displaying the superior intelligence to read this book.

The Push-Up

One of the oldest and simplest exercises known to man, the push-up is in a class by itself. Like the basic ab crunch, push-ups can be done anywhere, without any equipment. The downside to the push-up is that it uses your body for resistance, so as you get stronger and your body gets lighter, you'll have to do more of them.

Preparation

1. Get down on your hands and knees, and place your hands directly under your shoulders. The wider you put your hands, the harder this exercise is and the less your chest actually works, so keep them right at shoulder width. Using fancy push-up handles or doing fingertip push-ups does nothing to improve this exercise, so just a plain old flat hand on the floor is fine.

2. Stretch out your legs and put your feet right next to each other, or no more than a few inches apart. Your toes will be the only part of your body other than your hands to touch the ground, so be sure you are wearing good, solid athletic shoes.

3. The key to a proper push-up is keeping your body rigid. You want your entire body to move off the ground at one time. Try to maintain a straight line with your shoulders, your hips, and your feet. Don't let your hips sag like an old horse, and don't stick up your butt. Keep your body straight as a board.

Movement

4. Keeping your body straight, slowly bend your arms and lower yourself until either your chest comes in contact with the floor or your shoulders are lower than your elbows. Don't go down so far that you are lying on the floor; get close and then push back up again.

5. As you lower yourself, take a deep breath. Blow out this air as you are pushing up off the floor. Think of your breath as the fire coming out of a rocket that pushes the rocket off the ground.

Precautions

It may look cool, but adding weight on your back to increase the resistance of push-ups is a bad, bad idea that will only lead to injury.

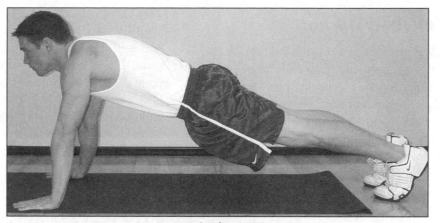

Starting/ending position.

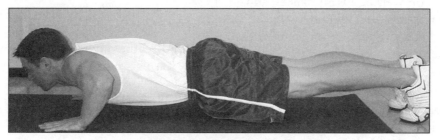

Midpoint position.

Modified Push-Up

It's totally okay if you can't start out with regular push-ups. In fact, only about 10 percent of the population can do more than one push-up. The modified push-up is for anyone who has trouble doing regular push-ups right off the bat. As you develop your pectoral muscles through modified push-ups, you'll eventually gain the strength you need to do regular ones. And that's what body sculpting is all about: building muscles gradually and safely to achieve the results you desire.

Preparation

1. Get down on your hands and knees, and place your hands directly under your shoulders. The wider you put your hands, the harder this exercise is and the less your chest actually works; be sure to keep them at shoulder width.

2. Your knees will be in contact with the floor, so it's a good idea to have an exercise mat or a carpeted surface under you. Put your knees together, cross one foot over the other, and lift your feet off the ground.

3. The key to a proper modified push-up is keeping your body rigid. You want your entire body to move off the ground at one time. Try to maintain a straight line with your shoulders, your hips, and your knees. Don't let your hips sag like an old horse, and don't stick up your butt. Keep your body straight as a board.

Movement

4. Take a deep breath as you bend your elbows and lower yourself toward the floor. Keep going down until either your chest touches the floor or your shoulders are lower than your elbows. Don't let your chest touch the floor, but come as close to it as possible.

5. Breathe out and push back up until your arms are straight again.

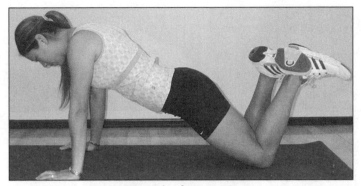

Starting/ending position.

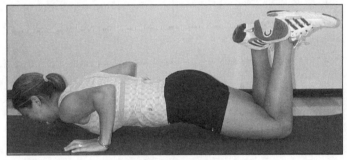

Midpoint position.

Stability Ball Push-Up

The stability ball push-up is an advanced exercise that will challenge you when you find regular push-ups boring (yes, you will get to the point that your sculpted muscles find some exercises too easy). The difference between the basic push-up and the stability ball push-up is that you have an unstable surface to push on. The ball will want to move around under you, so you will have to work even harder to keep it still. Also, instead of placing your hands under your shoulders, you'll extend them just a bit in front of you. It doesn't matter what size of stability ball you use, as long as it is at least as wide as your shoulders.

Preparation

1. Place your hands on the stability ball in a shoulder width position. If you can't get a good enough hold on the ball, let some air out of it. You don't want to end up kissing the ball because your hands slipped off.

2. Straighten out your legs and stiffen your body so you create a straight line from your shoulders to your hips to your feet. You will be up on your toes, so wear good, solid shoes.

Movement

3. Slowly lower yourself until you almost touch the ball. As you go down, inhale deeply.

4. While you exhale, push off the ball until your arms are straight again.

Precautions

◆ Most stability balls are burst resistant to prevent injuries, but they can puncture and deflate slowly. When using a stability ball, place it on a carpeted surface or exercise mat, in case you slip off the ball or the ball deflates.

◆ Without a stable surface under your hands, your wrists will move around a lot. If you have had wrist problems or issues with carpal-tunnel, you should forgo this exercise.

Variations

If you have a hard time keeping the ball still, try stabilizing the ball against two walls in a corner. The walls will prevent the ball from moving around, and you can master the exercise by first concentrating on the push-up portion of the exercise and working on the stability part later.

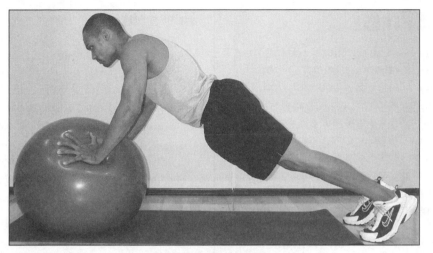

Starting/ending position.

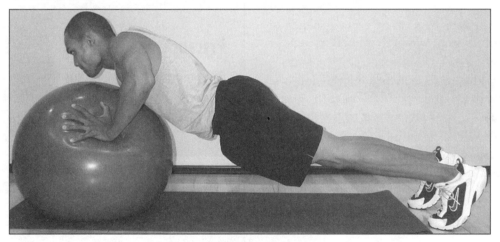

Midpoint position.

Dumbbell Press

The dumbbell press is an excellent exercise that allows you to work on your strength in combination with your balance and coordination. Lifting two weights can get a bit tricky, so start with a relatively light weight and get comfortable with the movement before tackling any heavy lifting. One of the key elements in the dumbbell press is balancing the weights so they move up and down together smoothly. We all have a dominant side that is a little stronger, so you may feel that one side of your body is not working as hard, but that's okay. With time, the dumbbell press will train your weaker side to catch up, and you won't be lopsided anymore.

Preparation

1. Lie on your back on an exercise bench or aerobics step, with a dumbbell in each hand.
2. Start the exercise by placing the dumbbells in a resting position on each shoulder, with your elbows out to the side, as shown in the photo.
3. Keep both feet on the floor, and keep your hips, butt, and shoulders on the bench.

Movement

4. Take a deep breath and, as you blow it out, press the dumbbells straight up over your chest until your arms are completely straight. Don't allow the dumbbells to hover over your head or down by your stomach. They should always be directly over your chest and shoulders.
5. Slowly lower the dumbbells back to your shoulders, breathing in as you lower them.
6. While the dumbbells are moving up and down, they should follow a straight, smooth path. If you see them moving out to the sides in a circular path to the top, bring them back in line. Moving the dumbbells out to the sides forces your biceps to work too much and uses extra energy.

Precautions

Anytime you have a weight over your head or chest, be sure to have a spotter. Don't do this exercise by yourself.

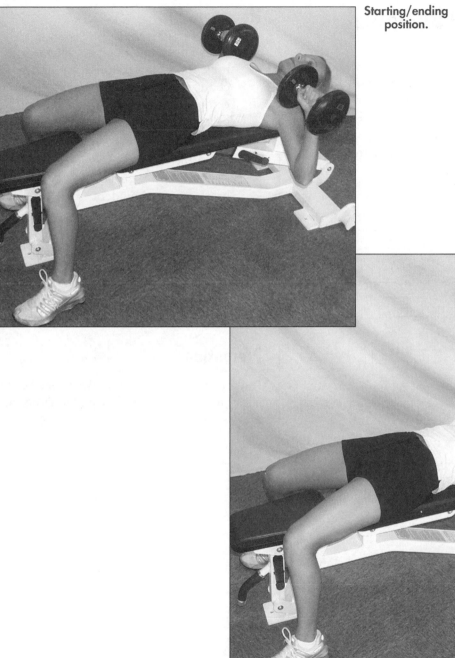

Starting/ending position.

Midpoint position.

Stability Ball Dumbbell Press

You can make the dumbbell press more difficult by using a stability ball instead of a bench. Using a ball takes away your stable base of support, so now your core and legs have to help keep you balanced while you move the weight. This is an advanced exercise, so get comfortable with the regular dumbbell press on a bench before you try it.

Preparation

1. Lie on the ball so it's directly under your shoulder blades. Because the ball is not very long, you will have to create a straight line from your shoulders to your hips to your knees to protect your back from injury. A wide foot stance will help keep the ball from rolling around, or you can move your feet closer together for more intensity.

2. Hold the weights next to your shoulders, with your elbows pointed out to the sides.

Movement

3. Take a deep breath and, as you exhale, press the weights directly up over your chest. Keep pressing until your arms are completely straight. You might feel the ball sinking a bit while you lift, which is normal.

4. Bring the weights together at the top of the press and then slowly lower them back to your shoulders.

5. The weights should move in a straight line up and down. If they are moving out to the sides or are jerking around, slow down and get them under control. If you can't move them up and down smoothly, reduce the amount of weight you're lifting.

Precautions

Anytime you have a weight over your head or chest, have someone spot you. Don't do this exercise by yourself.

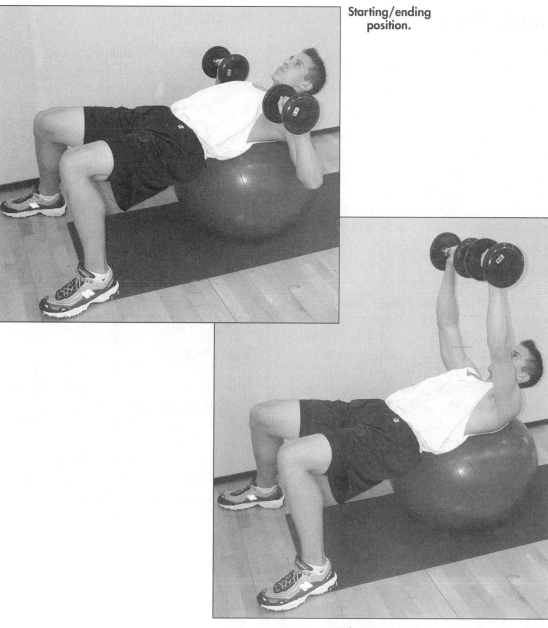

Starting/ending
position.

Midpoint position.

Dumbbell Fly

Unlike all the other "pressing" or "pushing" exercises in this chapter, the dumbbell fly does not use the triceps for help. Instead, this exercise provides good isolation for the pectorals only. The only downside is that you'll probably feel sore after exercising, so start easy and get used to the exercise before really packing on the weight. These photos show the dumbbell fly being done on a stability ball, which is an advanced move. If you don't have a ball, you can also perform the movement on a bench.

Preparation

1. Lie on the stability ball so it's between your shoulder blades and so your lower back and hips are extended in front of you. Create a straight line "bridge" from your shoulders, through your hips, to your knees, and hold it steady. Your feet can be placed as close together as is comfortable. The wider your feet are spaced, the easier the exercise is.

2. Start with the dumbbells positioned up, hovering over your chest and shoulders. The dumbbells should be touching and should never be over your head.

3. To prevent any elbow strain, bend your elbows slightly. Keep them "locked" in this position so they don't bend farther when you perform the exercise.

Movement

4. Inhale deeply, and slowly lower the weights to your sides, as if you were getting ready to hug a very big tree. Extend the weights until they are positioned just above your shoulders, as shown in the photo. You should still be able to see the weights out of the corners of your eyes.

5. Bring the weights back up to their starting point over your chest. Keep that "hugging" motion in mind so the weights will remain extended from your body. Keep the slight bend in your arms so the movement doesn't become a dumbbell press. As you squeeze the weight back up to the top, exhale.

Precautions

◆ This is another exercise that requires a spotter. Don't do this alone; we don't want any smashed noses from falling weights.

◆ Avoid extending your arms below shoulder level. This can cause elbow hyperextension and potential injury.

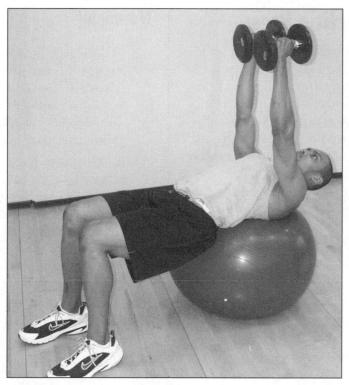

Starting/ending position.

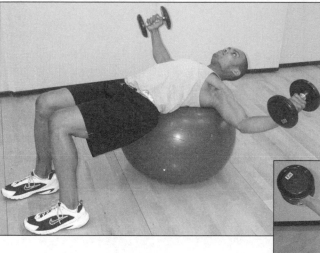

Midpoint positions.

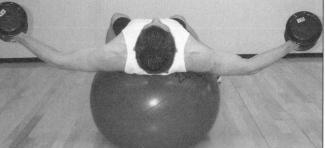

Dumbbell Incline Press

The dumbbell incline press is a first cousin of the regular dumbbell press. The difference between the two is that the incline press also works the front shoulder muscle (called the anterior deltoid). This won't fatigue the shoulder, and it is not a replacement for other shoulder exercises because the muscle isn't working to full capacity; it's working just enough that you'll notice. Another fun benefit of the incline press is that you can watch yourself doing it if you sit in front of a mirror. A mirror provides immediate feedback on your form and technique, plus you get to see those sculpted muscles moving around.

Preparation

1. Choose the degree of incline that's most comfortable. Most benches adjust from 15° to 75°. I suggest using somewhere around 45° so you can watch your progress in the mirror without getting too much of the shoulder involved (the steeper the incline is, the more the shoulder works).

2. Grab the dumbbells and have a seat. Do a small biceps curl to get the weights to the starting position just over your shoulders. Your elbows will be pointing out.

Movement

3. Take a deep breath and, as you exhale, press the dumbbells straight up over your chest and shoulders. Your arms will totally straighten as the dumbbells come together at the top. Again, don't let the dumbbells hover over your head.

4. Slowly lower the weights back to their starting point. Try to keep the weights moving in a straight line from your shoulders, up to the top, and then from the top back down to your shoulders. Any movement out to the sides makes your biceps work and wastes energy.

Precautions

This is another exercise that requires a spotter to keep you from dropping the weights in your lap.

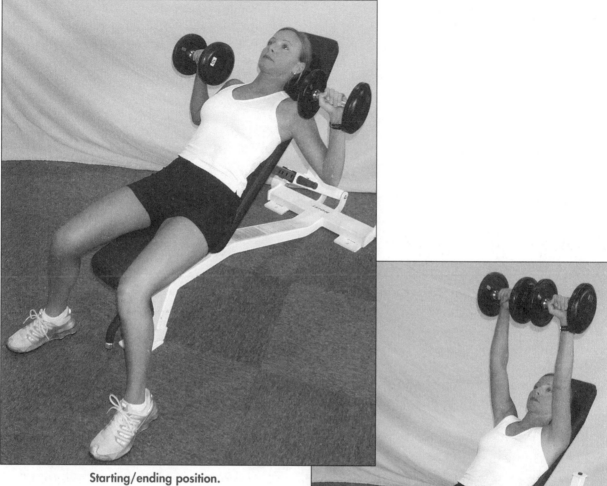

Starting/ending position.

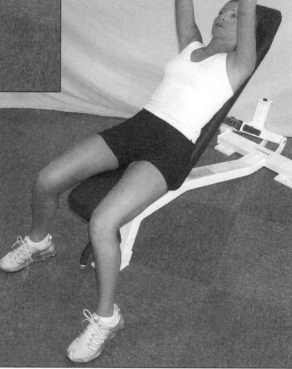

Midpoint position.

Machine Chest Press

Machines are excellent choices for working the chest muscles because you simply don't have to fiddle with balance and coordination. For those of you who are coordination impaired, or if you really want to isolate the chest muscles, machines are the best choice. The chest press machine goes by many names: vertical chest press, seated chest press, seated bench press, and as one of my clients likes to call it, "That hard one where you push out."

Preparation

1. Proper seat adjustment is the key to maximizing the effects of the chest press. Sitting too low or too high won't feel right and just plain looks funny. Imagine that a bar is running across your chest from each of the handles. Pretend that, instead of two handles, it's a solid bar. You want this bar to be at chest height, not neck height or stomach height. Adjust the seat up or down to achieve this position.

2. Most of the newer chest press machines have two sets of handles: a horizontal set and a vertical set. Ignore the vertical set, which are for another exercise. Grab the horizontal handles, and lift up your elbows so they are the same height as your hands. If you let your elbows hang down, you will force your shoulder muscles to do most of the work. You want to focus on the pectorals here, so lift those elbows high.

3. Sit up straight on the bench—no slouching. Keep your back flat against the pad and your feet flat on the ground.

4. Adjust your weight on the stack. Be sure to push the pin all the way in the hole, or the weights may come crashing down. (It won't hurt you, but it will make enough noise that everyone in the room will look at you.)

Movement

5. Take a deep breath, and exhale as you push the handles out. Keep pushing until your arms are completely straight.

6. Slowly lower the weight until the weights almost touch the stack, but not quite. You don't want the weights to come to a rest. Keeping the weight up a bit keeps your muscles working longer. Now just push it back out for another rep.

Variations

You can use machines to work one side of your chest at a time. Keep one hand in your lap, and go through the motions with one hand; then switch so you don't get lopsided results. By working one side at a time, you can focus on improving your weak side by doing a few more reps than with your strong side.

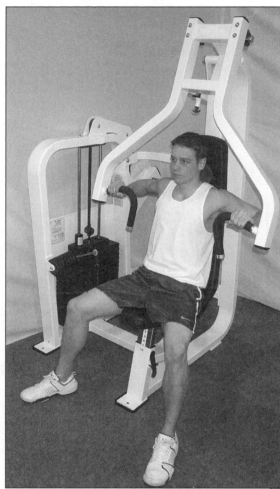

Starting/ending position.

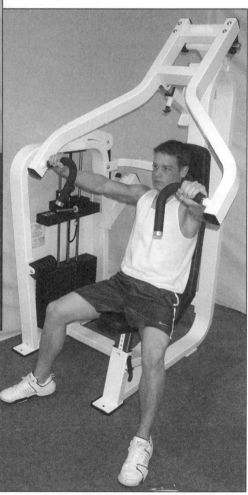

Midpoint position.

Machine Fly

The machine fly is a great exercise to watch in the mirror. I tell clients to pretend they are flexing their muscles like the bodybuilders on TV do. This exercise really shows off the definition you've been working so hard for, so enjoy the results.

Preparation

1. Adjust the seat to its proper height. As with the machine bench press, pretend there is a solid bar from one handle to the other. This bar should pass right across your chest. Adjust the seat up or down to achieve this position.

2. Depending on the brand of machine, you may also be able to adjust how far back the handles will go. If they're back too far, you can risk injury. But if they're not back far enough, you may miss out on part of the exercise. Adjust the handles so your hands are stretched out to your sides, but never farther back than your shoulders (any farther back puts your shoulder stability at risk).

3. Keep your arms straight, with just a slight bend in the elbows. This is not a pressing exercise, but a fly, so think big, long wings.

4. Sit up straight, and keep your feet on the floor.

Movement

5. Pretend you are hugging a giant tree. Maintain a slight bend in your elbows, and squeeze your arms together as you breathe out. This exercise is called a fly for a reason: Think about flapping your arms like a bird. Slowly bring your hands together far out in front of you.

6. When your hands meet, slowly return the weight to the starting position. Be sure not to let the weight completely rest on the weight stack before your next rep.

Precautions

You may feel a need to lean forward during this exercise. Don't. Keep your back flat against the pad, and keep your head out of the way of the arms of the machine.

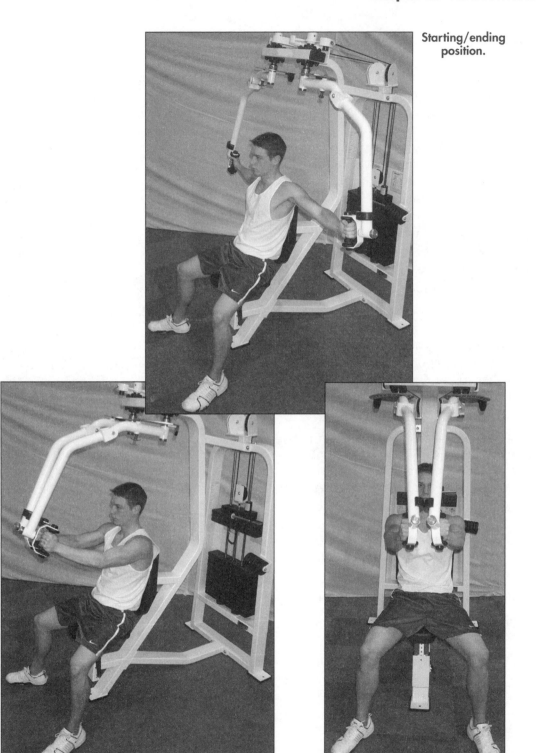

Starting/ending position.

Midpoint positions.

Bench Press

The renowned bench press is the granddaddy of all chest exercises. As one of the first organized exercises men competed in, the bench press continues to elicit a great deal of awe and envy to this day, particularly as the weights get heavier. Because each of the exercises in this chapter works the same muscles, the bench press doesn't have to be a fundamental part of your body-sculpting program. However, it's still a good exercise, so if you feel comfortable with it, here are some tips to maximize the movement.

Preparation

1. Lie down on the bench (on your back), and keep your feet on the floor. Some people like to put their feet on the bench, but that makes this exercise unstable and dangerous, so avoid this position.

2. Place your hands on the bar approximately shoulder width apart. Positioning your hands wider than shoulder width decreases the effectiveness of this exercise, and narrower will make the triceps work too much. Although there will probably be small marking rings around the bar, ignore them; they are for reference only.

3. Be sure your hands are an equal distance from the middle of the bar. You don't want to tip over.

Movement

4. Lift the bar off its resting hooks and hover it over your chest. Don't let it move over your head or down over your stomach. There is a point at which your arms will be perfectly vertical and the bar will feel relatively light.

5. Inhale deeply, and slowly lower the bar toward your chest. Keep the bar away from your head and neck! The bar also shouldn't come in contact with your chest—within an inch or so is fine.

6. While exhaling, push the bar back up until your arms are straight again. As you push, move the bar in a straight line. If you feel the bar moving more toward your head or stomach, make adjustments to keep it positioned over your chest.

Precautions

◆ Do not do this exercise without a spotter. It may seem funny on TV when someone gets stuck under a bar, but you definitely won't be laughing if it happens to you.

◆ Do not let the bar "bounce" off your chest. Some competitive lifters do this to get the bar moving upward, but it is really dangerous. Your chest is not a trampoline.

◆ Keep your back flat on the bench. Arching your back while pushing the bar up can strain your lower back muscles and cause injury.

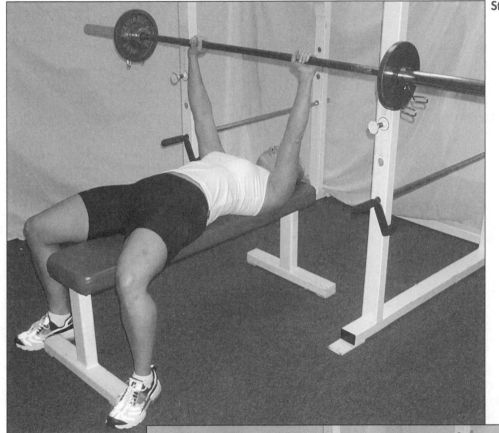

Starting/ending
position.

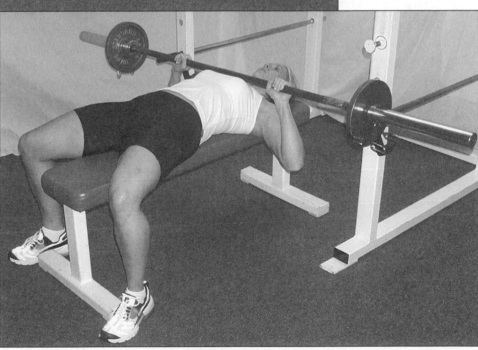

Midpoint position.

Tubing Press

You've gotta love resistance tubing. It bends, it stretches, and you can take it anywhere. It's a great way to work your chest if you don't have any heavy equipment and don't care to get down on the floor for push-ups. Tubing presses are a little different than the other chest exercises because the farther you stretch the tubing, the harder the exercise becomes. This is ideal for working the chest because you can actually handle more weight as your hands extend farther from you during the exercise. It's all about mechanical advantage and complicated physics. To put it simply: You are stronger near the end of the motion, so you can handle more weight there. Tubing does this naturally, so it provides a great way to work the chest.

Preparation

1. First, anchor the tubing by wrapping it around a pole, a doorknob, or something heavy that won't come flying at you when you pull on it.

2. Hold one end of the tubing in each hand, and face away from your anchor. The starting position for your hands is just under your shoulders, with your elbows out to the sides (pretend you're a chicken flapping your wings).

3. Put one foot in front of the other to create a solid base. As you push out on the tubing, it's going to try to pull you back. Positioning your feet solidly on the ground will keep you from moving.

Movement

4. Take a deep breath and then exhale while pressing out with both hands until your arms are straight.

5. Slowly bend your elbows and bring your hands back to their starting position near your shoulders. The tubing will try to pull you back quickly, so you will have to exert some force to allow your arms to return to the starting position without being yanked back.

Precautions

You can make this exercise more challenging by stretching the tubing farther from the anchor— but don't stretch the tubing any farther than you need to. If it's stretched too far, the tubing can snap like a rubber band and pop you a good one.

Variations

Do this exercise one hand at a time, if you like. Keep one hand next to your shoulder, and push out with the other. You can alternate left and right hands, or do a whole set with your left and then with your right.

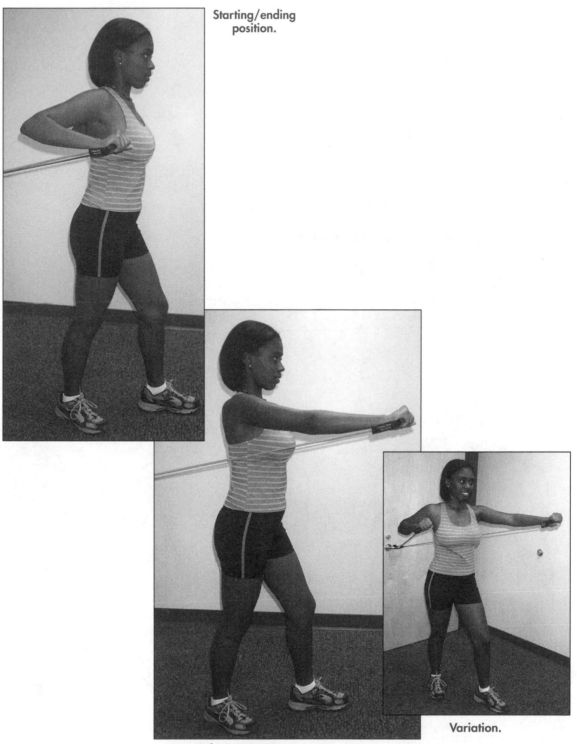

Starting/ending position.

Midpoint position.

Variation.

In This Chapter

- ◆ The importance of exercising your back
- ◆ Perfecting the pull-up
- ◆ Strengthening your lower back
- ◆ Upper back exercises
- ◆ Effectively using machines and tubing

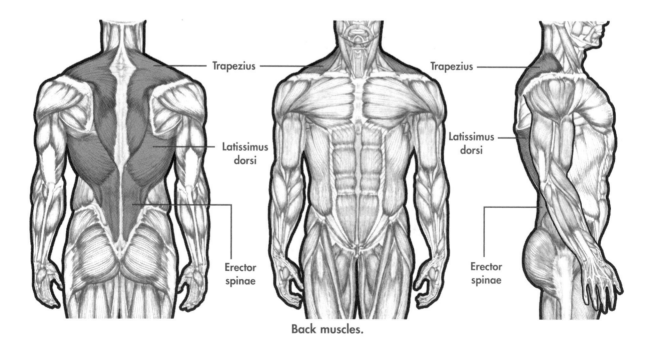

Back muscles.

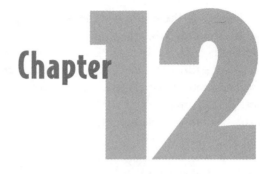

Chapter 12

We've Got Your Back

When you think of someone flexing his or her muscles, what do you see? Probably the front of the person: flexing biceps, chest, and abs. Because we tend to look into mirrors and see the front of our bodies, it's easy to forget that there are a bunch of muscles behind us that need attention, too. You can't easily appreciate back muscles by looking in the mirror, but they do look great on gals in low-back dresses and swimsuits, or on guys strutting their stuff at the beach.

Of course, it's important to work your back for more than aesthetic reasons. Your back muscles help balance the muscles of your chest and abdominals. Weak back muscles and strong chest muscles result in a hunched over, slouching appearance—not exactly a sculpted look. You don't want to end up like that, so balance your chest/ab workout with a healthy dose of back. In fact, most chiropractors will tell you that to prevent back pain, you should exercise your back regularly.

Lying Pull-Up

Fairly new on the exercise scene is the lying pull-up. All the kids are doing this one—literally. That's because the lying pull-up is part of the President's Physical Fitness Test. But just because kids are doing it doesn't mean you shouldn't. In fact, for the majority of adults, the lying pull-up is the only type of pull-up they can do. However, after working with lying pull-ups for a while, you will build up enough strength to handle regular pull-ups. Then you can tell all your nonsculpted friends that your muscle building is just child's play.

Preparation

1. This exercise requires a bar just high enough for you to reach while lying on the ground. I usually use a squat bar resting on the low hooks of a squat cage. Look around where you work out to find something similar.

2. Lie on the floor under the bar, and use a grip that's slightly wider than shoulder width. Adjust yourself on the floor so your arms are slightly angled toward your feet (about 20° or so).

3. Place your feet together, with the rest of your body lying stretched out. Think of this as the opposite of a push-up. At rest, you are essentially in the same position as the start/finish position of the push-up (except you're on your back).

Movement

4. Take a deep breath. As you exhale, pull yourself up until your chest reaches the bar. As you pull up, your entire body should leave the ground at one time. Pretend you are lying on a board that makes a straight line from your shoulders, through your hips, down to your feet.

5. Slowly lower yourself back down to the floor. You can actually rest on the floor between reps if you like (just try not to take a nap).

Precautions

To avoid falling from the bar, stop if you feel weak or if sweat is causing your hands to slip.

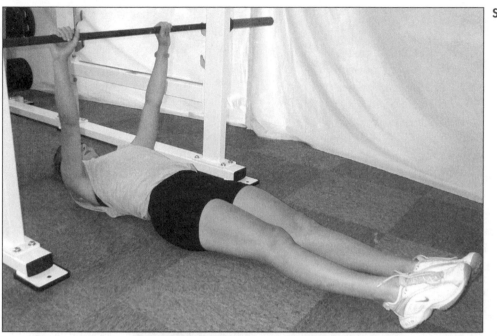

Starting/ending
position.

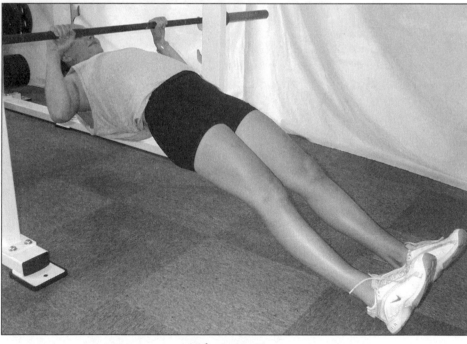

Midpoint position.

Pull-Up

Contrary to popular belief, there is a difference between a pull-up and a chin-up. The pull-up uses an overhand grip, whereas the chin-up uses an underhand grip. The small change in hand position completely alters the action of these exercises—in fact, they don't even look the same. (Turn the page to learn more about the chin-up.)

The pull-up is a great body-weighted exercise. It is also one of the most difficult exercises for beginners. The pull-up requires you to lift your entire body weight with each repetition. Unfortunately, when you're starting off, your body weight may be too much for your muscles to lift. But even if you can do only one or two reps, stick with it. Consistency is key, and a few reps every workout will quickly build into a full set.

Preparation

1. Find a pull-up/chin-up bar that's at least a couple inches higher than your reach. If you can reach the bar without jumping up to get it, be sure to bend your knees while doing this exercise. Otherwise, you will touch the ground each repetition, which will compromise the exercise's effectiveness.

2. Grab hold of the bar with a grip that's slightly wider than shoulder width. Most of the pull-up bars I've seen are much wider than anyone requires, so don't just grab the handles any which way; use the grip that's right for you. You will be using an overhand grip, with your palms facing away from you. See the close-up picture for clarification.

3. Hang from the bar in a completely relaxed state. (I like to hang from the bar just for the great stretch you get.)

Movement

4. Inhale deeply. As you breathe out, pull yourself up to the bar. Try to get your chin all the way to the bar (and no cheating by lifting your chin and stretching your neck!).

5. When you get to the top, don't stay and admire the view. Slowly lower yourself, and get ready for the next rep.

Precautions

During this exercise, be sure to lower your body slowly. Dropping quickly can overextend your elbows, which can be very painful.

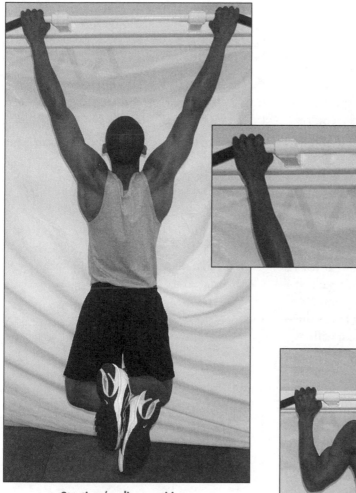

Starting/ending position.

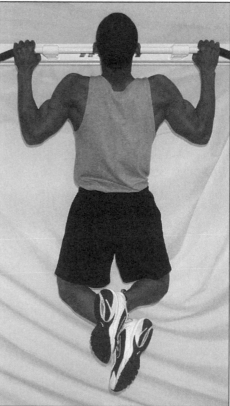

Midpoint position.

Chin-Up

The chin-up is the sister exercise of the pull-up. The only difference in technique is hand position and grip. These seemingly small variations, however, make the chin-up a great exercise for your biceps, too. And because you're using your biceps, the chin-up is usually much easier than the pull-up. If you've got strong biceps, you can probably do more repetitions of this exercise.

Preparation

1. Find a pull-up/chin-up bar that's at least a couple inches higher than your reach. If you can reach the bar without jumping up to get it, be sure to bend your knees during this exercise. Otherwise, you will touch the ground with each repetition, which will compromise the effectiveness of the movement.

2. Grab hold of the bar with a grip that's slightly narrower than shoulder width. You will be using an underhand grip, which means your palms should be facing you. See the photo for clarification.

3. Hang from the bar in a completely relaxed state (another great stretch).

Movement

4. Inhale deeply. As you breathe out, pull yourself up to the bar. You want to get your chin all the way to the bar (no cheating by lifting your chin and stretching your neck!).

5. When you reach the top, slowly lower yourself and get ready for the next repetition.

Precautions

◆ During this exercise, be sure to lower your body slowly. Dropping quickly can over-extend your elbows, which can be very painful.

◆ It will be really tempting to lift your knees, swing your legs, kick, and try to "climb" up the air. These movements will only waste energy and make your back work to stabilize your body rather than pull up to the bar. Always let your legs hang relaxed, and concentrate on pulling to the bar.

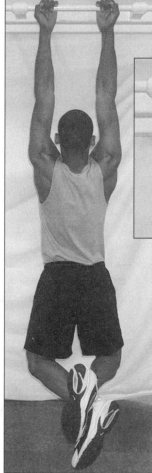

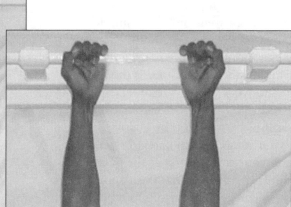

Starting/ending position.

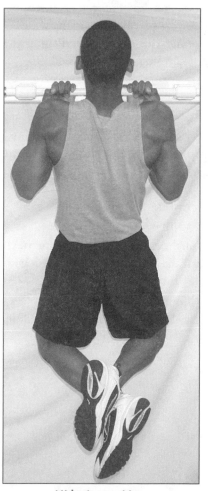

Midpoint position.

Extensions

If you asked me to pick my all-time favorite exercise, I'd say back extensions. It's a simple little exercise that produces huge results. Remember that the abdominals are considered the core of your body and that the core is the most important area to work? Well, the muscles in your lower back, called the erector spinae, make up the back half of your core. The abdominal muscles flex your torso, and the erector spinae muscles extend your torso. Look at the name erector spinae: It literally means "erect spine." When you see older people starting to hunch over, it's mainly because the erector muscles are weakening. A strong lower back helps keep you upright and strutting your sculpted stuff—plus, a strong lower back won't have as many aches and pains. Try doing this exercise first thing every morning when you get out of bed.

Preparation

1. Using the 45° extension bench (sometimes called a roman chair), adjust the thigh pad so it is just below your waist. You have to bend over the bench, so test it to be sure the pad is low enough that it doesn't hit you in the stomach.

2. Be sure your heels are set against the heel pads or heel plate that locks in your legs so you don't flip out.

3. Your legs should remain straight during this exercise. If you feel an uncomfortable pressure on your thighs, turn your toes out to the sides.

4. Cross your arms over your chest so they don't block your movement.

5. Slowly lower yourself by bending at the waist. Go as far down as you can. I've never seen anyone hit his or her head on the ground during this exercise, so just relax and let yourself hang.

Movement

6. Imagine a cat arching its back. Starting with your lower back, slowly lift yourself up by moving one vertebrae at a time. Roll yourself up slowly; do not keep your back flat and come up all at once. Your shoulders should be the last part of your back that unrolls. It may take practice to perfect this movement, but the results will be worth it.

7. As you unroll, come up only to the point at which your body is in a straight line. If you lift yourself any farther, you may hyperextend your back and cause injury. See the photos for the proper midway position.

8. Don't hold your breath. Keep breathing naturally through your repetitions.

Precautions

If you have back problems or pain, check with your doctor before starting this exercise.

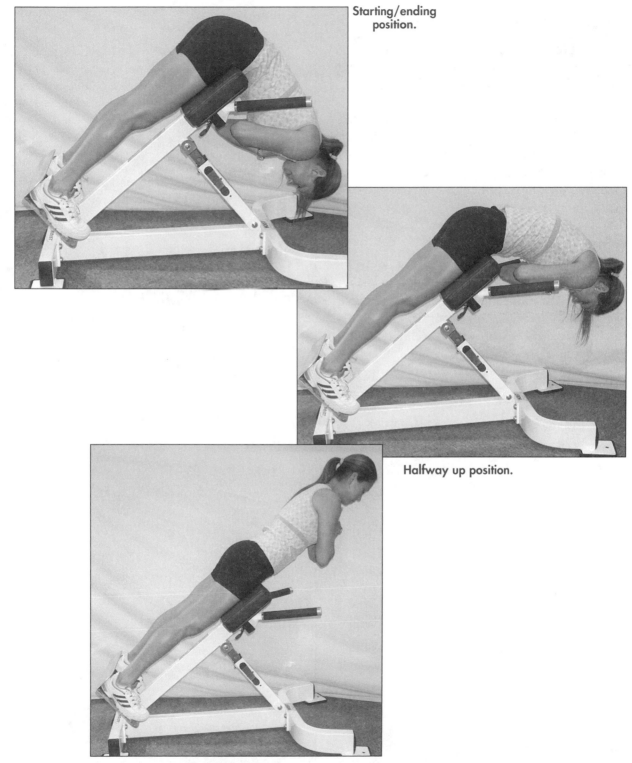

Starting/ending position.

Halfway up position.

Midpoint position.

Stability Ball Extensions

If you'd like to do a back extension, but your gym doesn't have the right bench, or if you want to do this exercise at home, use a stability ball to get the same effect. Use either a 45 or 55 cm ball; anything bigger will be difficult to lie across and have full range of movement. Be sure your ball is fully inflated and firm. If it flattens out too much when you lie on it, this exercise will be much more difficult.

Preparation

1. Lie across the ball so the top of the ball is positioned at your stomach. You may need to move the ball farther up or down to find a comfortable spot; you shouldn't have difficulty breathing. Relax and let yourself become one with the ball (a little zen to make things interesting). Your back should be arched in the same shape as the ball.

2. Place your hands on the sides of your head to keep them out of the way.

3. Extend your legs and balance on your toes. Your feet should be positioned widely enough to stabilize your position on the floor.

Movement

4. Starting with your lower back, slowly lift one vertebrae at a time. Unroll your body off the ball until you are completely straight. Your shoulders will be the last part of your back to unroll.

5. Slowly relax and lie back across the ball for the next rep.

6. Breathe naturally through your repetitions; don't hold your breath.

Precautions

If you have back problems or back pain, ask your doctor before starting this exercise.

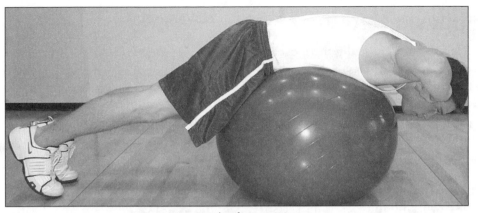

Starting/ending position.

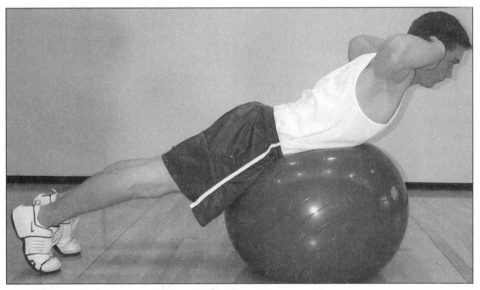

Midpoint position.

Lat-Pulldown Machine

The lat-pulldown is undoubtedly the most popular back machine in the gym. It also holds the distinction as the machine most improperly used. When used correctly, the lat-pulldown works the largest muscle in your back, known as the latissimus dorsi (or lats). This muscle reaches across most of your middle back and allows you to move your arms close to your body. Anytime you pull on something, the lats are the hardest-working muscles. This is also the muscle that gives your back a tapered look because it is wider at the top, narrowing as it travels down to your erector spinae.

Preparation

1. Find a lat-pulldown machine with a long bar attached to the cable. Grab hold of the bar at shoulder width using an overhand grip (palms facing away from you). No matter how wide the bar is, use only a shoulder-width grip—any wider will prevent you from completing a full range of motion.

2. Sit down in the seat, and place your knees under the pad. The pad gives you some leverage to help pull down the bar. For a more challenging move, don't use the pad (unless the weight you're lifting exceeds your body weight).

Movement

3. Starting with your arms completely straight, inhale deeply and pull down the bar in front of your head until it reaches your chin.

4. As you exhale, slowly let the bar back up. Let your arms stretch out completely before the next repetition.

Precautions

Never, ever pull the bar down behind your head! This is the biggest mistake I see in the gym. Some bodybuilder types will tell you that it makes the muscle contract more, but no scientific research supports that claim. Plus, pulling the bar down behind your head will eventually cause you shoulder and neck pain, and could cause injury.

Variations

As with the chin-up, you can switch to an underhand grip (palms facing you). Although the movement is the same—you'll pull the bar to chin level—this grip will allow you to also work your biceps, and you may be able to handle more weight.

You can also use a narrow V-grip bar. If you have wrist problems, the V-grip bar is easier because it places your hands in a neutral position (palms facing each other). Do the same movement, pulling the bar in front of you to chin level.

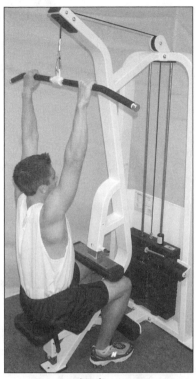

Starting/ending position.

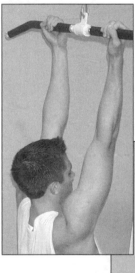

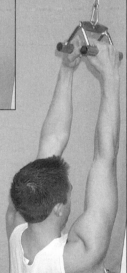

Variations.

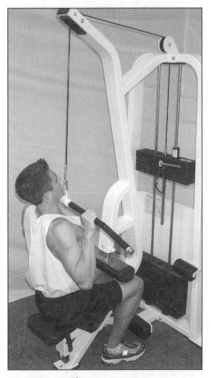

Midpoint position.

Seated Row Machine

Although the lat-pulldown is the most popular back machine, the seated row is probably the most useful for everyday life. After all, you pull objects in front of you much more frequently than you do those above you—like pulling the shopping cart backward because you just passed the refried beans, pulling your boyfriend or girlfriend in for a hug, or pulling open those heavy doors when the wind is blowing them shut. The seated row will help you do all this and more with greater effectiveness.

Preparation

1. Adjust the seat height so that when you grab the handles in a seated position, your arms are horizontal. Your arms should not be angled up or down to reach the handles.

2. Most seated row machines have two different handles—a horizontal pair and a vertical pair. Grab the horizontal pair.

3. Keep your elbows up and out to your sides, and keep your feet on either the floor or the foot rests (if the machine has them).

4. If the machine has a chest pad, using it is optional. It's actually more beneficial if you move back, sit up, and keep your back straight using your back muscles instead of the chest pad.

Movement

5. Inhale deeply. As you breathe out, pull back on the handles as far as you can. Try to pull your hands all the way back to your sides. If you can't get them that far, reduce the weight.

6. Slowly straighten your arms and release the bar back to the starting position.

Variations

Use the vertical grips. It's the same exercise, except your elbows stay down by your sides instead of being up and out.

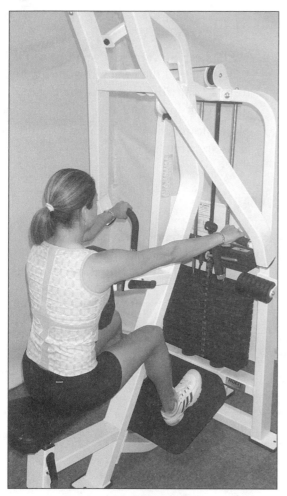

Starting/ending position.

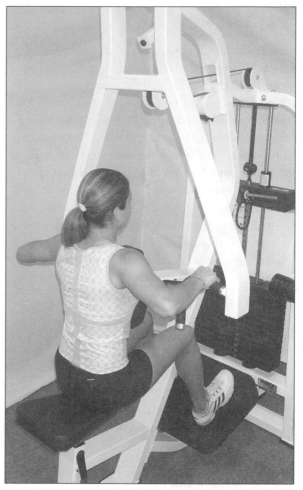

Midpoint position.

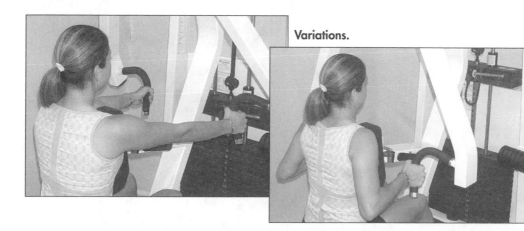

Variations.

Barbell Row

You probably do a version of this exercise all the time without even realizing it: Picking up your kids' toys and clothes, moving boxes, carrying laundry up two flights of stairs, and even taking out the trash qualify. So why do more? You probably already know the answer to that: The more weight and the more reps, the more sculpted your body will be. This exercise is especially good because it tones your upper back while strengthening your lower back. Plus, most back injuries occur when people are picking things up off the ground without a strong lower back; this exercise will help prevent that.

Preparation

1. Grab hold of a barbell or EZ-curl bar with a shoulder-width grip.
2. Bend your knees slightly, and also bend at the waist about 45°–60° (see the photos for clarification). Keep your back straight; slouching can cause you to injure your lower back.
3. Relax your arms, and let them hang straight down.

Movement

4. While keeping your back straight and still bent over, pull the bar up toward the bottom of your ribs. Try to get the bar to touch your lower chest.
5. Slowly lower the bar back down until your arms are straight.

Precautions

◆ Pay close attention to your lower back. Don't let it round during this exercise. Keep it straight by contracting those lower back muscles.

◆ Don't jerk the weight up. Pull it slowly. The only part of your body that should be moving is your arms. If you are raising your entire body during the movement, you're using momentum instead of muscle, and you won't get an effective workout.

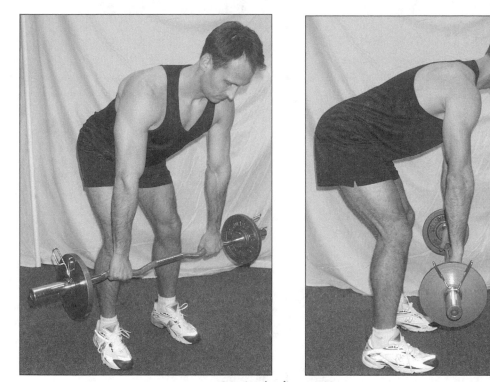

Starting/ending position.

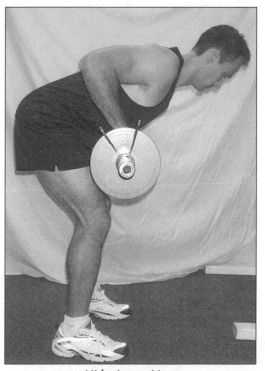

Midpoint position.

Dumbbell Row

If you don't feel comfortable with the barbell row, or if you have some lower back problems, the dumbbell row is a good alternative. This exercise requires using only one arm at a time, with your body stabilized on a bench, so your back is at less risk. This exercise also allows you to focus on each side of your back individually. Most of us have one side that is a little stronger, which is usually the same side as your dominant hand. With this exercise, you can isolate each side to get them evenly sculpted.

Preparation

1. You do this exercise one side at a time. Start with your right side. Spread your feet apart, and put your left foot about two feet in front of the right. Put your left hand on your left knee.

2. Hold the dumbbell in your right hand, with your arm hanging straight down and relaxed.

3. Bend at the waist, keeping your back flat and straight. You have to bend only about 30°–45°, just enough so you are pulling the dumbbell up to you. If you have a mirror, watch yourself and keep an eye on your back muscles.

Movement

4. Pull the dumbbell up toward the bottom of your ribs, lifting your elbow high. Try to get your hand all the way up to the side of your body.

5. Slowly lower the dumbbell and repeat for more reps.

6. After a set on the right side, switch sides. Put your right hand on the right knee, and hold the dumbbell in your left hand. Now do your left set.

Precautions

As I mentioned, keep your back flat. I see a lot of people lifting the dumbbell and their shoulder at the same time. It's awkward and wrong. The only part of your body that should be moving is your arm.

Starting/ending position.

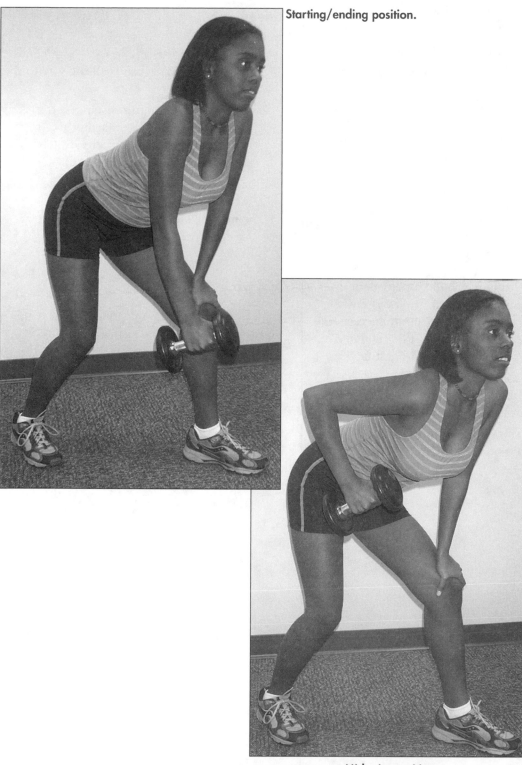

Midpoint position.

Tubing Row

The tubing row is different from all the other back exercises because, as you stretch the tubing, the exercise becomes more challenging (and when it comes to body sculpting, challenging is a good thing). This is another back exercise you can do just about anywhere. Even a pull-up/chin-up requires a strong bar to hang from, but for the tubing row, all you need is a piece of tubing. You can take this one with you when you travel.

Preparation

1. Wrap the tubing around a pole, door-knob, or something that won't move when you pull on it (your husband in the recliner might be a good option). The tubing should be situated at about chest height.

2. Grab one end of the tubing in each hand. Hold your arms straight out, and step back until the tubing starts to stretch.

3. Stand up straight, and put one foot behind the other for better balance.

Movement

4. Pull back on the tubing with both hands. Try to bring your hands all the way to the sides of your body.

5. If there isn't enough resistance—that is, if it's too easy—step back farther to stretch the tubing (remember, more stretch equals a more difficult exercise).

6. Slowly let your arms back out. The tubing will try to pull you forward, so keep your back straight and your feet in place for support.

Variations

You can also do this exercise with one arm at a time, either a full set on each arm or alternating arms with each repetition.

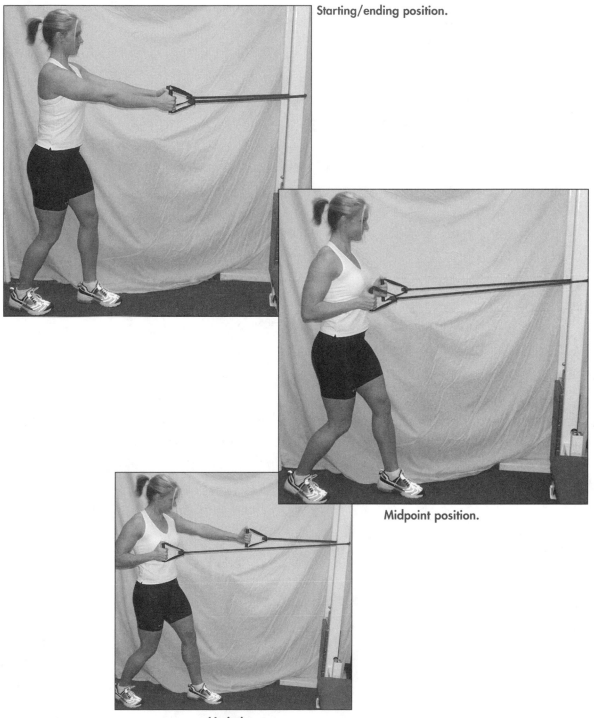

Starting/ending position.

Midpoint position.

Variation.

In This Chapter

◆ The benefits of strong, sculpted shoulders

◆ Targeting the different parts of the shoulder

◆ Using dumbbells and barbells safely and effectively

◆ Using machines and tubing to work your shoulders

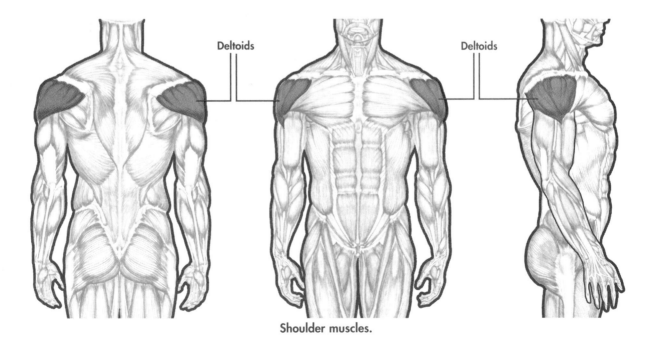

Deltoids   Deltoids

Shoulder muscles.

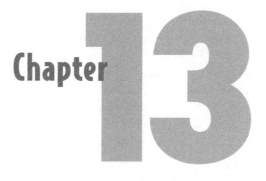

Shoulder This Challenge

Just below your neck, on the top of each arm, reside muscles you couldn't move your arms without: your deltoids. The deltoid muscles are typically divided into three portions: front, middle, and rear deltoid. Responsible for coordinating the movements of your arms, your shoulder muscles simply don't get the resistance-training respect they deserve—until now. Want sculpted shoulders to show off that new sleeveless dress, or strong and broad shoulders to fill out your new suit? Then pay some special attention to the exercises that isolate these important muscles.

Of course, every exercise that involves the arms, chest, or back also involves the shoulders, mainly as a stabilizer. But these exercises don't work the shoulders to the extent they really need. Spend some time isolating these workhorses, and you can have the kind of strong, well-defined shoulders that really stand out in a crowd and make a great place to hang your coat.

Dumbbell Lift

The dumbbell lift works all your shoulder muscles at the same time and even gets your biceps involved. In fact, anytime you pick up something off the floor to put on a counter, get the groceries out of the trunk, or pull up your pants in the morning, you are mimicking the dumbbell lift. I call this the "pick me up" exercise because it's exactly what you do to pick up a small child. So if you don't have kids around to act as your weights (or if you do and you want to have the strength to lift them more easily), try this simple exercise to sculpt the roundness of your shoulders.

Preparation

1. Hold a dumbbell in each hand, with your palms facing your legs.
2. Stand with your feet slightly apart for balance.

Movement

3. Imagine there are strings tied to your elbows and that someone is pulling on the strings. Your elbows should lift up, and the dumbbells should follow.

4. Bring the dumbbells right up under your chin, without actually hitting yourself (don't laugh, this actually happens). Keep the dumbbells close together. When you finish, your elbows should be higher than your wrists.
5. Slowly lower the dumbbells back down in front of you.

Precautions

Don't yank the weight up too quickly; you really do risk hitting yourself in the chin. Also, if you let momentum take over, you compromise the intensity of your workout.

Variations

You can also do this exercise one arm at a time. If you choose to go the one-arm route, avoid leaning over when you lift. Keep your body straight, and lift your elbow straight up. Your other hand should be holding a dumbbell in front of you for balance.

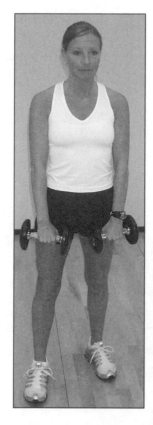

Starting/ending
position.

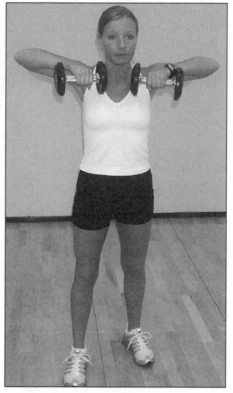

Midpoint position.

Dumbbell Front Raise

Dumbbells are about the best tool to use for your shoulders because they allow your arms to move independently of each other. Some trainers suggest doing this exercise with both arms at the same time, but I think it's more effective to concentrate on and isolate one shoulder at a time. This exercise isolates the front portion of your deltoid the most, which is the part you primarily use for everyday tasks such as picking up things and reaching out. Try doing this exercise in front of a mirror; you'll really be able to see the definition with each repetition.

Preparation

1. Stand with your feet slightly apart for balance. If you stand with your feet together, you will end up swaying back and forth as you lift the dumbbells. Also, place one foot in front of you and the other foot behind you, for a good, solid stance.

2. Hold a dumbbell in each hand, with your palms facing your legs.

Movement

3. Start with one arm, and slowly lift the dumbbell straight out in front of you. Your arm should stay as straight as possible.

4. Raise the dumbbell until it's at eyeball level—*your* eyeball, that is. You can probably go higher, but it's not really necessary; you've already done the hardest part of the movement.

5. Slowly lower the dumbbell back to your leg, and repeat with the other arm, alternating back and forth.

Precautions

If you risk hyperextending your elbow (that is, if your elbow can naturally bend backward a bit), be sure to keep your elbow slightly bent when lifting the weight.

Starting/ending position.

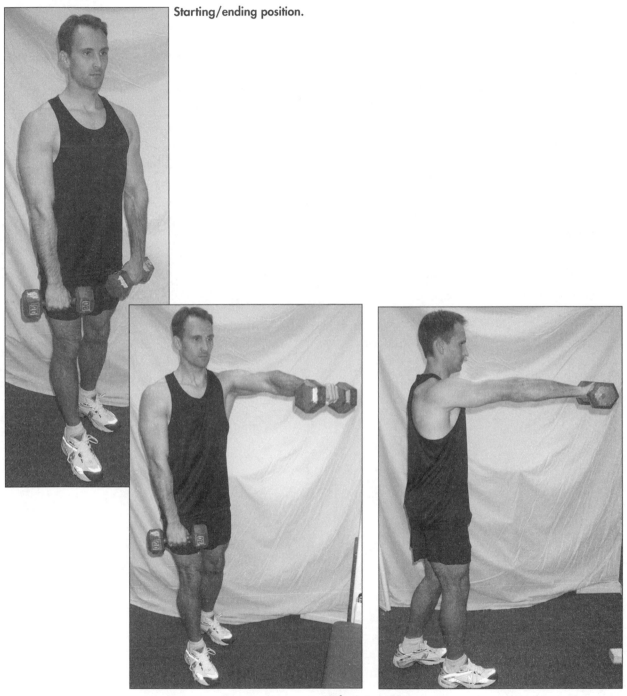

Midpoint position.

Dumbbell Lateral Raise

This isn't a movement you'll do in everyday life very often, but it's definitely one of the best ways to build the tops of your shoulders. The lateral raise really targets the middle portion of the deltoid—the part that runs across the top of your shoulder and down toward your biceps. Don't worry about your shoulders getting too big; this exercise will give them more definition without a lot of bulk.

Preparation

Find an area free of obstacles in which do this exercise. Because you'll be lifting your arms out to your sides, you'll want to avoid smacking objects or, worse, other people.

1. Stand with your feet apart, one foot slightly behind the other for balance.
2. Hold a dumbbell in each hand against the outside of your thighs, palms facing your legs.

Movement

3. Keeping your arms straight or just slightly bent at the elbow, lift both arms out to your sides until the dumbbells are at shoulder height.
4. Slowly lower them back to your sides. You may be tempted to simply let your arms drop, but you'll lose half the effectiveness of the exercise by neglecting to work your muscles on the way down, too.

Precautions

◆ You must do this exercise with both arms at the same time. A one-arm lateral raise unnecessarily strains your lower back.

◆ If you feel any shoulder pain, or if you have been diagnosed with shoulder impingement, lift the dumbbell only as high as you can without experiencing pain. Don't "work through" the pain; this may lead to additional injury.

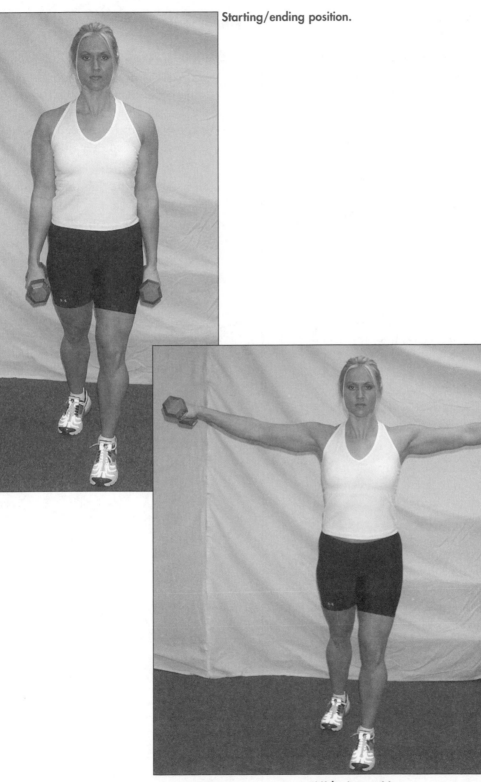

Starting/ending position.

Midpoint position.

Dumbbell Press

The dumbbell press can be performed sitting on a bench, perched on a stability ball, or standing up. That means, no matter where you are, you can do this exercise. The dumbbell press combines a full shoulder exercise with a bit of triceps training. I often use the dumbbell press with older clients who have trouble reaching over their heads to do everyday tasks such as getting things off a high shelf. This exercise helps strengthen their muscles so they can regain movement. By doing this exercise when you're young, you'll develop this strength now.

Preparation

1. If you choose to do this exercise seated, sit on the ball or bench with your legs apart so you have a good, balanced stance. If you have trouble keeping your back straight, or if you tend to slouch, use a bench or chair with a back rest that you can lean against. Or do the exercise standing.

2. To do the exercise standing, spread your feet for good balance. For even better balance, put one foot behind the other.

3. Hold a dumbbell in each hand and lift both to shoulder level, placing them either in front of your shoulders or to the sides of your shoulders, whichever is more comfortable.

Movement

4. Press both dumbbells up over your head at the same time. If the dumbbells naturally move together at the top of the lift, that's okay. Press up until your arms are completely straight. Keep a good grip on the dumbbells so they do not sway forward or backward.

5. Slowly lower the dumbbells back to your shoulders.

6. As you lift the dumbbells up and down, envision them moving along a nice, straight line. Allowing them to sway forward or backward only wastes energy.

Precautions

◆ If you have any back problems, forgo this exercise. Keeping your spine erect while lifting can place great strain on your back.

◆ Because you are lifting a weight over your head, be sure to use a spotter for this exercise.

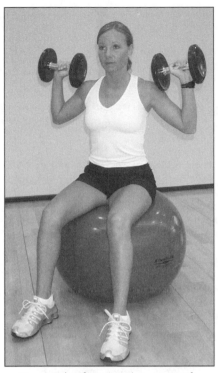

Starting/ending position—seated.

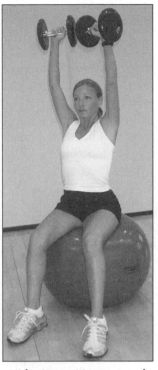

Midpoint position—seated.

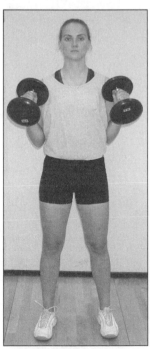

Starting/ending position—
standing.

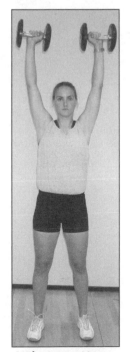

Midpoint position—
standing.

Barbell Lift

This exercise is similar to the dumbbell lift, except that you use both shoulders at once to lift a single object: the barbell. This movement is particularly useful if one shoulder is a bit weaker than the other. The strong shoulder can help the weaker one with the lift, and, as a result, the weaker muscle will be able to complete more repetitions. With time, your weaker shoulder will catch up to the stronger side.

Preparation

1. Stand with your feet apart, with one foot slightly behind the other, for good balance.

2. Hold the barbell against your thighs, using an overhand grip (palms facing toward your legs) just narrower than shoulder width. This is one of the only times you will use a grip this narrow, but in this case, it'll prevent your wrists from bending too much at the top of the lift.

Movement

3. Keep your elbows out to the sides and higher than the bar, and pull the bar up in front of your body until it's directly under your chin. Don't do the movement too quickly or you'll risk hitting your chin with the bar—not a pleasant experience, I can assure you.

4. At the top of the lift, your elbows should be higher than your wrists, and your wrists should be higher than the bar.

5. Slowly lower the bar back down the front of your body until your arms are completely straight again. You can let your shoulders sag a bit to stretch them, if you like.

6. For you gals, you will have to lift the bar out and around your breasts. Keep the bar as close to your body as you can when you do.

Precautions

◆ Keep your back straight, and don't allow your body to sway during the exercise. If you find yourself hunching over the bar (you'll know if you do this because the bar will hit you in the chest before it reaches your chin), stand up straight or use a lighter weight.

◆ If your wrists bother you during this exercise, use a dumbbell lift instead.

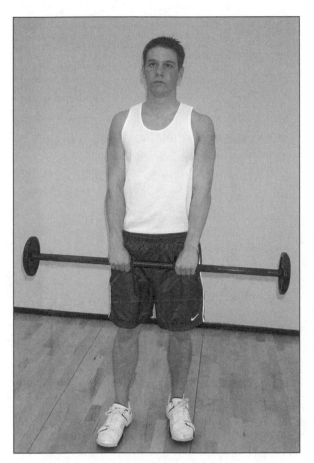

Starting/ending position.

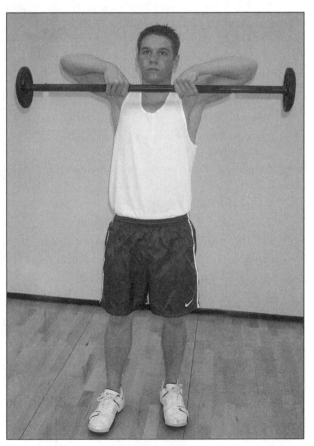

Midpoint position.

Barbell Raise

The barbell raise works the front of the shoulders while strengthening the lower back, which acts as a stabilizer. Both shoulders are working in synch during the barbell raise, but the movement can still be pretty difficult. Whenever you lift both arms out in front of you, the weight causes your center of gravity and center of balance to move forward. To compensate for this, you have to lean back a little, which makes your lower back work very hard. If your shoulders aren't very strong, your back has to work even harder. Because this exercise isn't meant to work your back, try to build shoulder strength with the dumbbell front raises and barbell lifts outlined earlier in this chapter before you attempt this exercise.

Preparation

1. Stand with your feet apart, with one foot slightly behind the other. Be sure you feel very steady and balanced.

2. Hold the barbell down against your thighs with an overhand grip (palms facing your legs). Be sure to use a strong grip, or you risk dropping the barbell (watch out for toes!). Your hands should be exactly shoulder width apart.

Movement

3. Keep your back straight, and don't let your body sway or swing back and forth. Concentrate on allowing only your shoulders to do the work.

4. With your arms straight or just slightly bent at the elbows, lift the bar out in front of you until it is at shoulder height.

5. Slowly lower the bar back to your thighs. Be sure not to drop it quickly because you want to work your shoulders on the way down, too.

Precautions

It's very easy to get in a bad habit of swinging the weight up, using momentum instead of muscle for the movement. Be sure to concentrate on maximizing the use of your shoulders for this exercise.

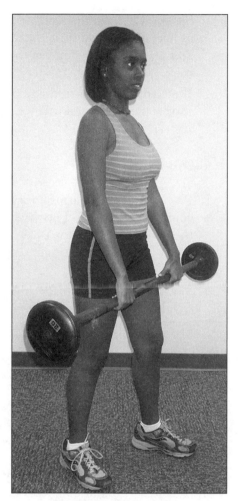

Starting/ending position.

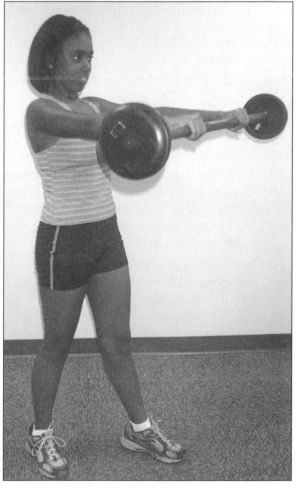

Midpoint position.

Machine Shoulder Press

The shoulder press machine is a great way to work all the front, middle, and back portions of your shoulders at one time. The shoulder press machine is also a good alternative to the dumbbell press if you don't have a spotter available. The direction the machine travels is preset, so you don't have to worry about balancing the dumbbells or ensuring that both arms are in synch. All you have to do is provide the pushing power, so it's nearly impossible to do this one wrong (unless you sit on the machine backward, which I don't advise).

Preparation

1. Adjust the seat on the machine so that when you sit down, the handles are right next to your shoulders. If the seat is too high, it will be difficult to grip the handles and probably impossible to lift. If the seat is too low, you won't experience a full range of motion, and the exercise won't be as effective.

2. There are usually two sets of handles, one set pointing at you and one set pointing out in front of you. It doesn't matter which set you use; just be sure to use the same handle on each side.

3. Sit up straight in the seat. Keep your back as flat as possible during the movement. You may feel that you need to arch your back, but don't; keep it flat.

4. Place your feet flat on the floor, with a wide stance, for good balance.

Movement

5. Push up with both arms until they are completely straight. The machine guides the handles, so you don't have to worry about them going the right way—there is no wrong way.

6. Slowly let your arms back down until the weight stack almost touches and then push back up. If you allow the weight to rest, you take all the work off your shoulders and the exercise is less effective.

Precautions

As I said previously, be sure to keep your back straight! If you can't lift the weight without arching your back, lighten the weight. Arching your back hyperextends your vertebrae, a position that will lead to lower back pain.

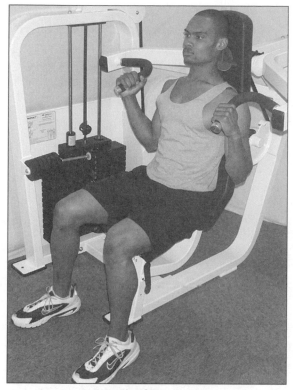

Starting/ending position.

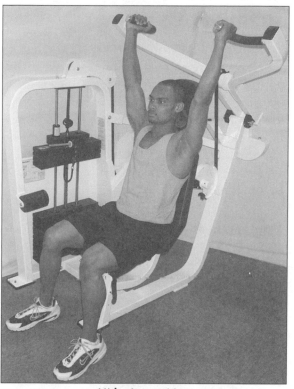

Midpoint position.

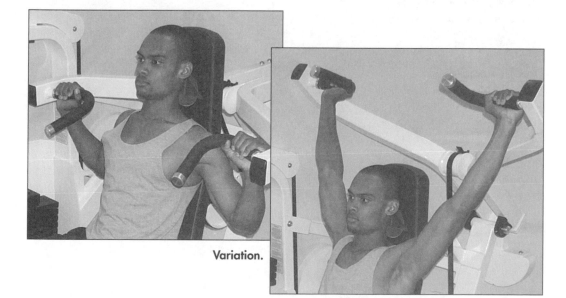

Variation.

Tubing Press

The tubing press is another way of working shoulders using an overhead movement, without the need of a spotter. Using tubing is great because, as you stretch it, the exercise becomes more difficult. Tubing provides a specific advantage when working your shoulders because, as you reach higher, your shoulders actually get stronger—and that's just when the tubing press becomes more challenging.

Preparation

1. Stand with your feet slightly apart, with one foot in front of the other.

2. Place the middle of the tubing under your front foot. Concentrate on applying most of your weight to your front foot—it's no fun if the tubing slips out and pops up toward your face.

3. Hold the ends of the tubing in each hand, with your palms facing forward. Your hands should be right next to or just above your shoulders.

Movement

4. Simultaneously press both hands up toward the ceiling until your arms are as straight as possible. Don't allow your hands to sway forward or back. At the top of the movement, your hands should be directly over your shoulders.

5. Slowly lower your hands back to your shoulders. Because tubing is just a big rubber band, and you've really stretched it out, it will naturally try to spring back down quickly. Control the descent, and bring your hands back to where they started.

Precautions

Because you are stretching the tubing quite far, be sure your shoes don't have any sharp edges that could cut the tubing, and ensure that the tubing is not torn anywhere. An unexpected snap into your body isn't the most pleasant experience.

Always keep your back straight. Don't lean back more than you would if you were just standing—and don't lean forward, either.

Variations

You can also do this exercise one shoulder at a time. Start in the same position, with both hands next to your shoulders, but do the movement with only one hand—and one shoulder—at a time. Alternate hands for a balanced workout.

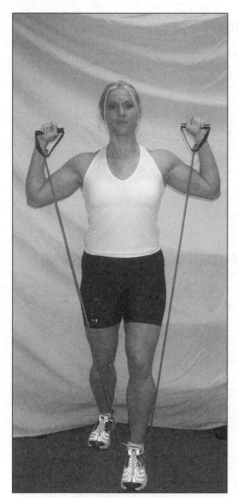

Starting/ending position.

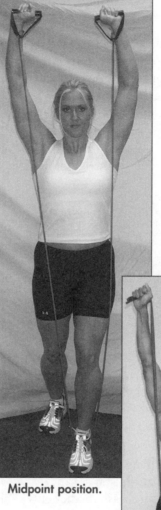

Midpoint position.

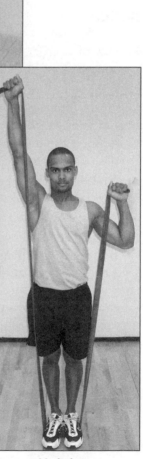

Variation.

Tubing Raise

The tubing raise is almost exactly the same as the dumbbell raise, except the resistance increases as the tubing stretches, which makes this exercise potentially more difficult. Don't let that scare you off, though. The shoulders are weakest at the top part of this exercise, so the additional resistance will really stimulate the muscles to work and become stronger as well as more sculpted.

Preparation

1. Stand with your feet slightly apart, with one foot in front of the other.
2. Place the middle of the tubing under your front foot. Concentrate on applying most of your weight to your front foot—it's no fun if the tubing slips out and pops up toward your face.
3. Grab hold of each end of the tubing. Your arms should hang down in front of you, with your palms facing your legs.
4. The tubing should now be stretched a bit. If the tubing is lying slack, you won't have any resistance at the start of the exercise, which will decrease the benefits you get from the movement. You may have to wrap the tubing around your foot once to take up some slack.

Movement

5. Keep both arms straight or just slightly bent at the elbows. Lift your hands in front of you until your hands are at shoulder height, keeping your palms facing down toward the ground.
6. Slowly let your arms back down, while controlling the stretch of the tubing. Keep those muscles working in both directions.

Precautions

You might feel like you need to lean back, but don't. Keep yourself standing straight, with no leaning or swaying.

Variations

You can also do this exercise one arm at a time. Isolate one shoulder by doing several reps in a row, or alternate left and right.

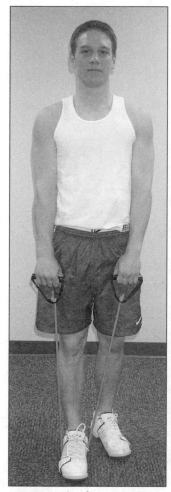

Starting/ending position.

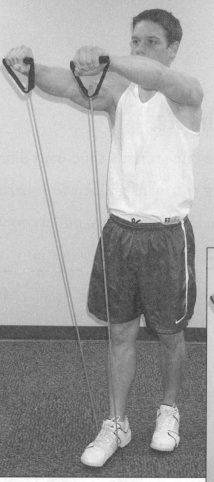

Midpoint position.

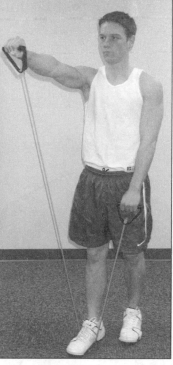

Variation.

In This Chapter

◆ Isolating one arm at a time with dumbbells

◆ Working two arms at once with barbells

◆ Using machines and low-pulleys to work your biceps

◆ Maximizing your biceps workout with tubing

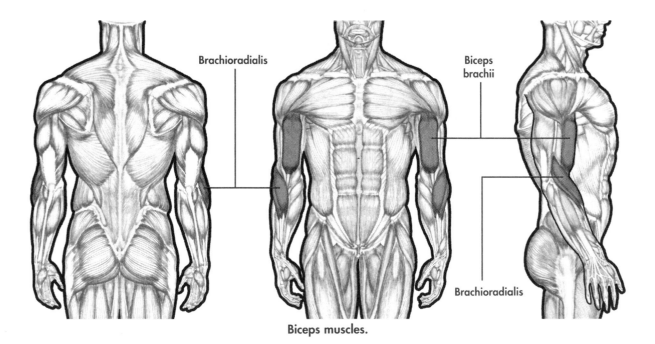

Biceps muscles.

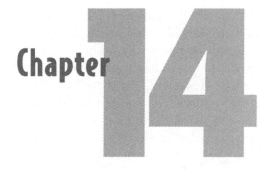

Chapter

Armed with Buff Biceps

When you tell people you're on a body-sculpting program, they're bound to ask at some point to see your muscles. The classic answer is to roll up your sleeve, flex your biceps, and wow them with the definition and strength that characterizes your arm. Of course, it may take a little time, but that's what this program is all about.

The biceps have always been given special attention in the world of bodybuilding and physique contests, and now you, too, can have the kind of arms that make people think, "That person is definitely in shape." The main job of your biceps is to bend your elbow, so all the exercises in this chapter involve just that—usually with some sort of weight attached. Your biceps are also used in many of the back exercises in Chapter 12. And of course, you use your biceps in vitally important everyday activities—just try bringing your fork up to your mouth without bending your elbow!

Dumbbell Curl

The dumbbell curl is probably one of the main reasons dumbbells were invented. Dumbbell curls provide one of the best methods of isolating one arm at a time, by applying direct resistance to the biceps. The dumbbell curl (and any biceps exercise with an underhand grip) works both the biceps brachii and the brachioradialis muscles, known collectively as the biceps. Try to do this exercise in front of the mirror, where you can see the muscles working and monitor your form.

Preparation

1. Stand with your feet apart and a dumbbell in each hand. Both dumbbells should weigh the same, even if you have one arm that's stronger. Unequal dumbbells will result in unequal results—you'll be lopsided.

2. Hold the dumbbells with an underhand grip (palms facing away from you). Let the dumbbells rest against the outside of your thighs. You arms should be completely relaxed, but not so relaxed that you drop the weights.

Movement

3. To keep from leaning back, perform the dumbbell curl with one arm at a time. (Leaning can strain your back.)

4. When lifting, keep your elbow at your side. The only part of your body that should move is your forearm and hand. Smoothly pull the dumbbell up to your shoulder by bending your elbow.

5. When you get to the top of the curl, slowly lower the dumbbell back to rest beside your leg. Your arm should be completely straight and relaxed. Alternate arms, allowing one arm to rest while the other is working.

Precautions

The biggest mistake I see people making with dumbbell curls is swinging the weight. You may believe that you're "lifting" more, but you're actually letting momentum do the work for you, making the exercise less effective. Don't swing.

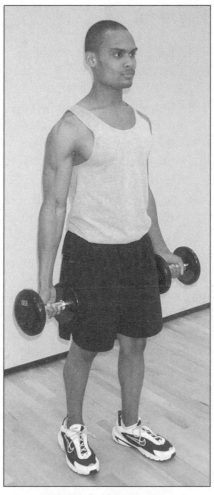

Starting/ending position.

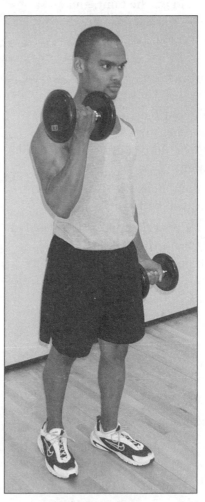

Midpoint position.

Hammer Curl

With this exercise, you hold the dumbbell as you would a hammer and then move your arms as if you're hammering a nail—hence the name hammer curl. Hammer curls work the same muscles as the dumbbell curl. Because of the way the arm is held, you won't see as much "flexing" during a hammer curl, but don't worry: You will still get a sculpted result. If you have any elbow problems (such as tennis elbow), hammer curls are a good alternative to dumbbell curls, which can cause pain in a problem elbow. They put less strain on the joint, and most of my clients who do this exercise say they prefer it over dumbbell curls.

Preparation

1. Stand with your feet apart, and hold a pair of dumbbells in your hands. The dumbbells should rest against the outside of your thighs.
2. Hold the dumbbells with a neutral grip. Your palms will be facing your legs.
3. Keep your arms relaxed at your sides. Do not flex or bend your elbows.

Movement

4. Keep one arm at rest beside you. This exercise works one arm at a time to protect your back from unnecessary stress.
5. Pull the other dumbbell up to your shoulder by bending your elbow. Your elbow should remain at your side when you lift the dumbbell; only your forearm and hand should move.
6. Slowly let the dumbbell back down to your side, and repeat with the other arm.

Precautions

Pay attention to where the weight is at all times. I've had clients actually hit themselves in the face with the dumbbell when they curl it up. And as with the dumbbell curl, avoid using momentum to lift the weight—don't swing.

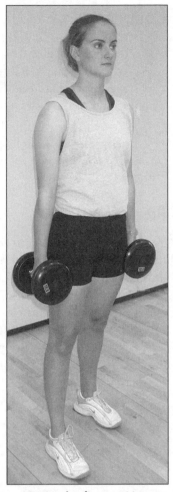

Starting/ending position.

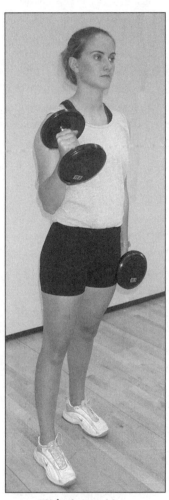

Midpoint position.

Concentration Curl

Concentration curls get their name because you have to concentrate on completing a set with just one arm at a time, while keeping the strictest of form. A concentration curl is a bit more difficult than other dumbbell curls because you are concentrating all your effort on one little muscle group that's being worked over and over without any rest. The upside is that this exercise makes the biceps work more, and the results often show it. It's also an ideal exercise for helping a weaker arm catch up to a stronger one. Because you are working one arm at a time, you can do a few extra reps or an extra set for the weaker arm until both arms have equal strength.

Preparation

1. Sit on the end of a bench, or on a stool, chair, or stability ball.

2. Spread your feet wide apart; you will be doing this exercise between your legs.

3. Place your left hand on your left knee for support while you work your right arm (switch this to work your left arm).

4. Hold the dumbbell with an underhand grip (palm facing away from you), and let the dumbbell hang down inside your leg.

5. Bend over at your waist—keeping your back straight—and let your elbow rest against the inside of your leg, right next to your knee.

Movement

6. Bracing your elbow against your leg, bend your elbow and curl the weight up toward your shoulder. Don't let the dumbbell hit you in the face.

7. Slowly lower the dumbbell until your arm is completely straight and then repeat until you finish the set.

Precautions

You might feel like you need to lean back or to the side to lift when you start getting tired. Don't do this. Be sure to keep your back straight during the whole exercise. You want to focus your effort on the biceps muscles, and leaning is a form of cheating that will decrease your results. The only parts of your body that should be moving are your forearm and hand.

Starting/ending position.

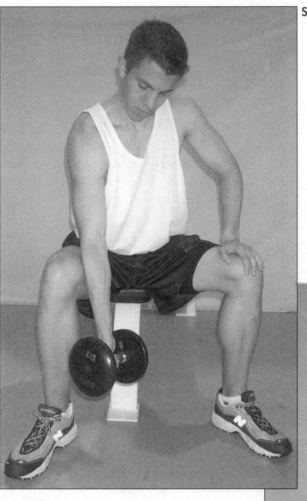

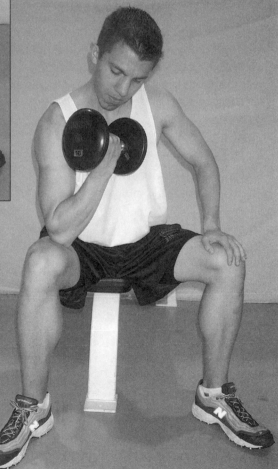

Midpoint position.

Barbell Curl

If dumbbells aren't your thing, or if you want to work both arms at the same time to save time, head for the barbell rack. A barbell provides the same emphasis on the biceps muscles as the dumbbell curl, but because it keeps the wrists in a locked position, the movement provides even greater benefits to both the biceps brachii and the brachioradialis. Barbell curls really make your biceps flex and stand out, so do these in front of a mirror and check out your sculpting results firsthand.

Preparation

1. Stand with your feet apart, with one foot slightly behind the other. You really need a solid base of support while doing this exercise because the lifting movement will make you want to lean back. Be sure to keep your back straight for proper form.

2. Hold the barbell in both hands using an underhand grip (palms facing away from you). Your grip should be about shoulder width, evenly spaced from the center or ends of the bar. Let the barbell rest against the front of your thighs.

Movement

3. Keep your body still and your elbows at your sides. Bend both elbows, and curl the barbell up to your shoulders. Both sides of the barbell should reach your shoulders at the same time, so curl with a steady, balanced movement.

4. Slowly lower the barbell back to your thighs, and relax your arms before the next repetition.

Precautions

As I mentioned, this exercise will make you want to lean back, but resist the temptation. Leaning back won't make the exercise any easier, and it could hurt your back. Be sure to stand up straight.

Variations

If your wrists get sore from holding a barbell, use what's known as an EZ-curl bar. Instead of being straight like a barbell, the EZ-curl bar is bent so it's wavy. It's easier on the wrists and accomplishes the same goal, so use it if you need to.

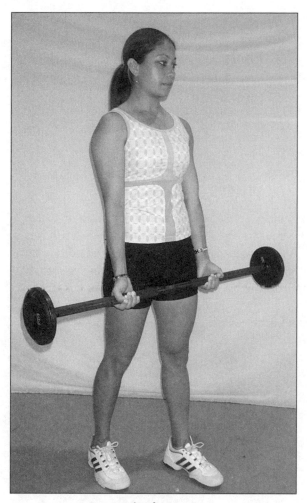

Starting/ending position.

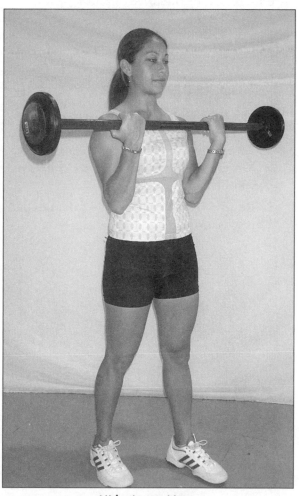

Midpoint position.

Overhand Curl

Any time you use an overhand position (your palms face down instead of up) with a biceps exercise, you make your forearms work harder because they are responsible for maintaining your grip. But how does this benefit the biceps? Many of my clients cannot do a full set of bicep curls because their grip is weak and they cannot hold on to the dumbbell or barbell. Overhand curls help you improve your grip while also exercising the biceps—you really do get two exercises for the price of one.

Preparation

1. Stand with your feet apart, with one foot slightly in front of the other.
2. Hold the barbell with an overhand grip (palms facing down or toward your legs). Your grip should be evenly placed on the barbell, slightly wider than shoulder width.
3. Rest the barbell against the front of your thighs, arms relaxed.

Movement

4. Keep a very tight grip on the barbell, and keep your elbows next to your sides.
5. Curl the barbell up to your shoulders.
6. Slowly lower the barbell back to rest on your thighs (maintaining a tight grip).

Precautions

This exercise is designed to strengthen your forearms so you can do more biceps exercises. When your forearms become fatigued, your grip weakens. If your grip weakens, you could drop the barbell. So as soon as you get tired and fear you might drop it, finish your set. Rest a bit before you start another set.

Variations

You can do this exercise with dumbbells, if you like. Use the same movement, but work one arm at a time. That way, you can concentrate on the grip even more.

Starting/ending position.

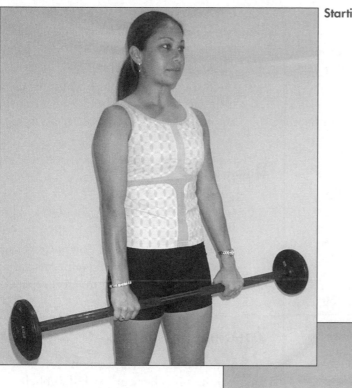

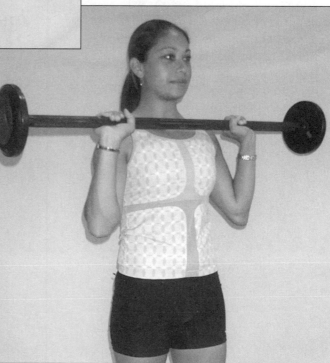

Midpoint position.

Preacher Curl

You don't have to say a prayer during this exercise, but it never hurts. The preacher curl uses a special bench that provides your arms with a place to rest. This creates a more stable position for your arms than when you are holding weight beside you without any support. The extra support and stabilization give you the ability to focus on your biceps without worrying about keeping strict form—meaning it's tough to mess this one up.

Preparation

1. Adjust the height of the seat or the arm pad, depending on the model of bench. You want to sit comfortably, with your upper arm flat on the padding. If your elbows are the only part of your arm touching the pad, you are sitting too high, so lower the seat. If your elbows can't touch the pad, but the top of your arm near your armpit touches it, you are sitting too low, so raise the seat.

2. Use either a regular barbell or an EZ-curl bar. The EZ-curl bar has become the standard on the preacher curl, so that's what's shown in the photos.

3. Hold the bar at shoulder width or just a little narrower than shoulder width using an underhand grip (palms facing up).

Movement

4. Curl the bar up to your shoulders. The bench will help you keep proper form.

5. Slowly let the bar back down. Lower the weight completely until your arms are straight before starting the next repetition.

Variations

To isolate and concentrate on one arm at a time, do the preacher curl with dumbbells. Hold one dumbbell over the bench just as if you were using a barbell, and let the other hand rest.

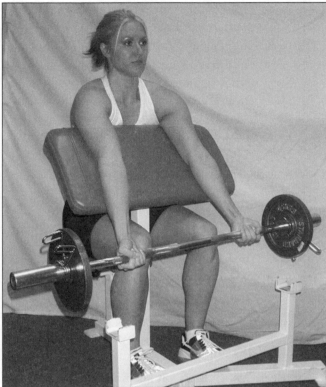

Starting/ending position.

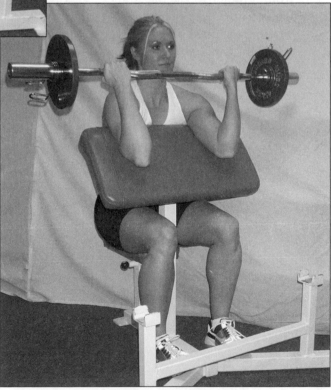

Midpoint position.

Low-Pulley Curl

Pulley machines are becoming more prevalent in health clubs and gyms. Many of the new styles of biceps machines use pulley systems with interchangeable handles that allow you to do different types of biceps exercises (such as one-hand vs. two-hand curls). A distinct advantage of pulley machines over dumbbells and barbells is that the resistance remains consistent throughout the range of motion. With dumbbells and barbells, there is very little resistance at the midway point of the exercise, so the low-pulley curl can give you a sculpting advantage.

Preparation

1. Low-pulley machines have a number of different handle attachments to choose from. I prefer to use the straight bar for biceps curls because it gets both arms working together, which saves time. Attach a straight handle bar to the low-pulley cable.

2. Grasp the handle with an underhand grip (palms facing away from you). The grip placement depends on how wide the handle is. Use a close grip with your hands only a few inches apart, or a wider grip that spans your shoulders (but never wider than your shoulders).

3. Hold the bar down in front of you, letting your arms relax.

4. Stand back about a foot from the low pulley. Spread your feet apart, and put one foot in front of the other for good balance. When you do the low-pulley curl, you will feel as if you're being pulled forward. Having a good stance will prevent you from falling into the machine.

Movement

5. Keeping your elbows at your sides, curl the bar up to your shoulders.

6. Slowly lower the bar until your arms are straight again.

Precautions

Really concentrate on keeping your body from leaning backward or forward. Leaning may compromise the effects of the exercise and could even lead to injury.

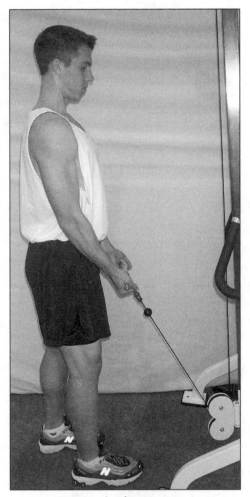

Starting/ending position.

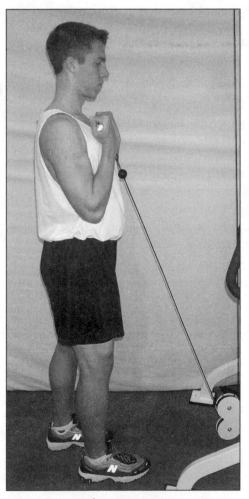

Midpoint position.

Biceps Curl Machine

The biceps curl machine is a great alternative to the preacher curl, utilizing the same movement with a weight stack/machine mechanism instead of free weights. The benefit of using a machine over free weights is that a machine has a set range of motion, so you can move in only one direction. Plus, it makes both arms work together; one arm can't get ahead of the other. The overall advantage of using a machine is that you don't have to worry about form as much, and you'll work the biceps just as hard as with free weights, providing that elusive "burn."

Preparation

1. Adjust the height of the seat or the arm pad, depending on the model of bench. Your goal is to sit comfortably, with your upper arm flat on the padding. If your elbows are the only part of your arm touching the pad, you are sitting too high, so lower the seat. If your elbow can't touch the pad, but the top of your arm near your armpit touches it, you are sitting too low, so raise the seat.

2. Grasp the handle no wider than shoulder width with an underhand grip (palms facing up).

3. Adjust where your elbows rest on the machine so that both you and the machine pivot at the same point. There should be some kind of hinge or axis where the handle is attached to the machine. Line up your elbows with this pivot point so you are working *with* the machine, not against it.

Movement

4. Keep your elbows in that pivot point, and curl the bar up to your shoulders. Because the machine controls your range of motion, you're not likely to compromise form.

5. Slowly lower the handle, being sure to straighten your arms completely before starting the next repetition. If the weight stack touches (there isn't any resistance) before your arms are completely straight, adjust either the seat or the alignment of your elbows.

Precautions

Don't "bounce" your arms when you lower them. This can strain your elbow tendons or sprain the elbow ligaments, neither of which is any fun.

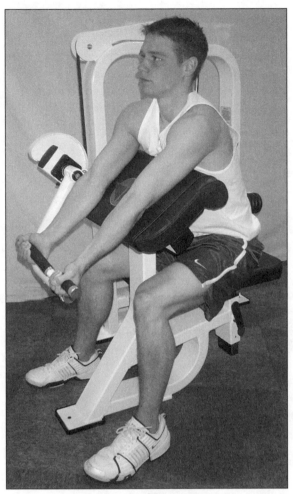

Starting/ending position

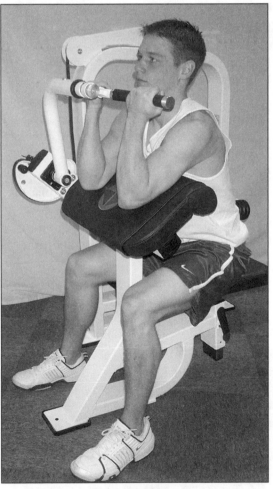

Midpoint position.

Tubing Curl

The tubing curl is very effective because it becomes increasingly difficult as you perform the rep. Unlike curls with dumbbells and barbells that get easier near the top of the movement, or low-pulleys that have the same level of difficulty throughout, tubing curls really challenge the muscles as the exercise goes on. You can adjust the resistance simply by moving the foot that anchors the tubing, and you can perform the exercise with either one or two arms at a time.

Preparation

1. Stand with your feet apart, one foot in front of the other.
2. Hold the ends of the tubing in each hand using an underhand grip (palms facing up). Keep your arms relaxed and down at your sides.
3. Place the center of the tubing under your front foot. To anchor the tubing, place it under the arch of your foot. If it's too near the toe or heel, it could slip out. Place most of your body weight on the front foot.

Movement

4. To work both arms at the same time, keep your elbows at your sides and curl the tubing up to your shoulders. Remember, it's going to get more difficult as the tubing stretches, so keep pulling and don't give up.
5. Slowly let the tubing back down. Unbend your elbows until your arms are again relaxed at your sides.

Variations

Instead of exercising both arms at once, alternate one arm at a time or complete an entire set on one arm, followed by the other. When isolating one arm, keep holding the tubing in the other hand for support and balance.

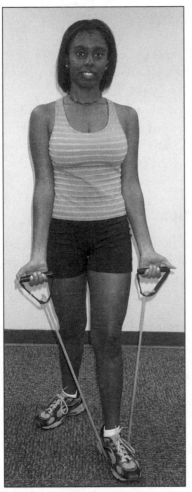

Starting/ending position.

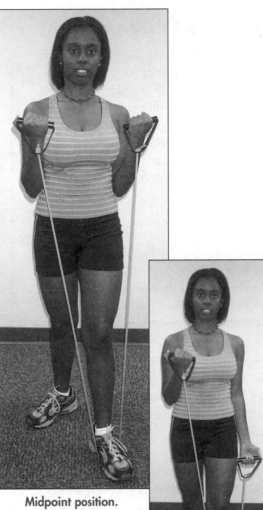

Midpoint position.

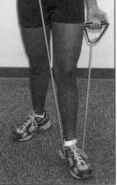

Variation.

Seated Ball Tubing Curl

The seated version of the tubing curl provides a greater challenge by incorporating an unstable surface beneath you. Not only will your biceps work to curl the tubing, but your core muscles also will work to keep you balanced on the ball. This exercise is best performed on a very firm stability ball, but you can also use an office chair that has wheels for a similar effect.

Preparation

1. Sit on the top of the ball, feet in front of you. The closer together your feet are, the more difficult this exercise is; however, don't place your feet too wide because your arms have to work outside your legs. If you're using a chair, sit on the very edge, but be careful not to slip off.

2. Hold the ends of the tubing in each hand. Place the center of the tubing under the center of both feet. Be sure to apply some weight to your feet so the tubing doesn't slip out.

3. Start with your hands at your sides, palms facing up (underhand grip). The tubing should have a little bit of stretch in it at this point (some resistance is good to start with).

Movement

4. Keeping yourself steady on the ball, with your elbows at your sides, curl both hands up to your shoulders.

5. Slowly lower your arms until they are straight and relaxed. The tubing will want to snap back quickly, so try to control the movement.

Variations

You can do the exercise one arm at a time, either alternating hands or completing a full set on one arm and then the other.

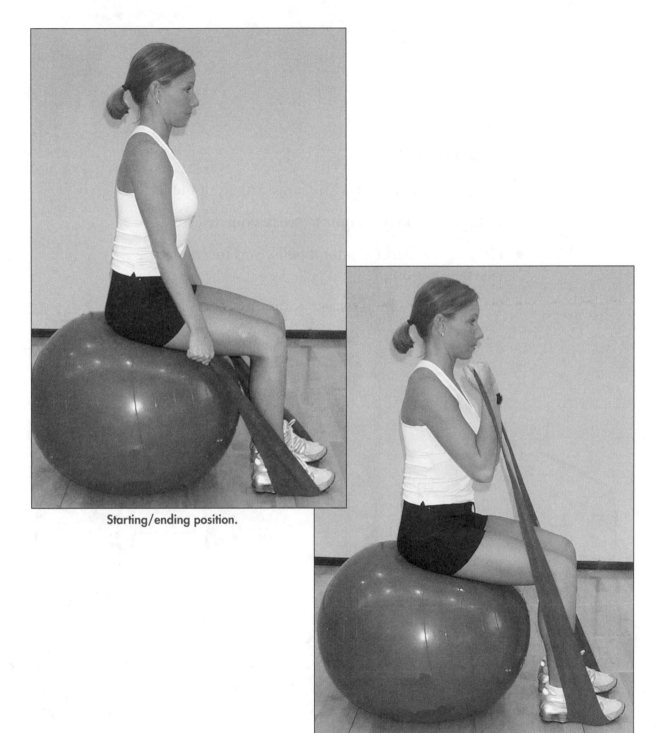

Starting/ending position.

Midpoint position.

In This Chapter

◆ Working the triceps without special equipment

◆ Using your body weight to work your triceps

◆ How to use barbells, dumbbells, and tubing for triceps sculpting

◆ Cable and machine triceps training

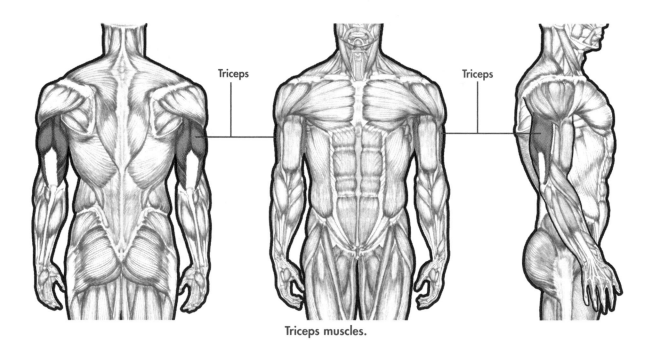

Triceps

Triceps

Triceps muscles.

Chapter 15

Triple Threat Training: Triceps

What's the hardest-working muscle in your arm? If you said the biceps, I'd have to disagree. My answer is actually the triceps. Why? Anytime you perform a pressing or pushing movement with the chest or shoulder muscles, the triceps help complete the motion. The exact opposite of the biceps, the triceps' job is to extend, or straighten, your elbow. So your triceps really do a lot of work they don't get credit for.

The triceps area of the arm is often a trouble area, particularly for women. Fat and flab tend to collect there, particularly if this area isn't given the attention it deserves. The good news is that you can gain a lot of definition and really sculpt your arms by isolating the triceps muscles with exercises designed just for them.

Seated Dip

Anytime you push yourself out of a chair or off the couch, you are actually doing a small version of the seated dip. The great thing about the seated dip exercise is that it requires no special equipment; you can use a chair, a bench, a stool, an aerobics step, or your couch for this exercise. That also means you'll never have an excuse for skipping it! Seated dips are a good beginning exercise to prepare you for vertical dips as well—covered later in this chapter, they are a bit more challenging.

Preparation

1. Find a flat bench, a chair, an aerobics step, or even your couch. Whatever you choose to use, be sure it is stable enough that it doesn't tip over or slide when you push down on the edge of it.

2. Sit on the edge of the bench with your hands on the bench right at your sides, fingers pointing toward your feet.

3. Holding yourself up by your arms, scoot your butt off the edge of the bench and slide your feet out in front of you until you have made a "bridge" out of your body. You'll need to use your lower back muscles to keep your butt from sagging toward the floor. The goal is to make a straight line from your shoulders to your feet.

Movement

4. Slowly let your elbows and hips bend, as if you were going to sit down on the floor.

5. Lower yourself until your shoulders are at the same level as your elbows and your upper arms are parallel to the floor. If you end up sitting on the floor, either you've gone too low or your bench isn't high enough.

6. Push on your hands to straighten your arms, and tighten up your lower back to straighten your body to the starting position.

Precautions

If you've ever dislocated your shoulder, or if you experience any shoulder pain while performing this exercise, do not continue. Try another triceps exercise in this chapter as an alternative.

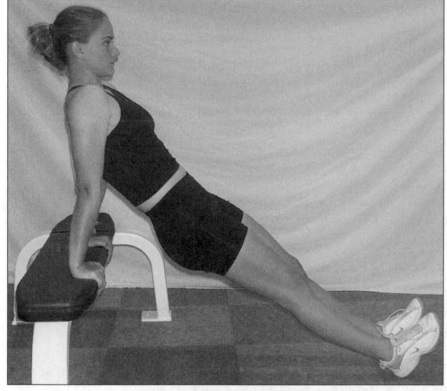

Starting/ending position.

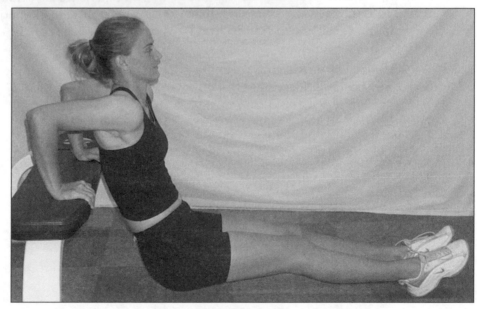

Midpoint position.

Vertical Dip

The vertical dip is an exercise that utilizes your body weight to isolate the triceps. Vertical dips, which really give the triceps a good "burn," fall into the same category as push-ups and pull-ups. Because they use your entire body weight, they are particularly difficult. Vertical dips become less challenging as you reach your body-sculpting goals, however. Because you're using your body weight as resistance, as you become lighter and stronger, the movement gets easier. This exercise is also sometimes referred to as simply a dip.

Preparation

1. Use a dip stand specially made for doing vertical dips. A dip stand usually is combined with a hanging-leg raise stand or a pull-up stand; ask your fitness center staff where you can find it.

2. Typically, the arms of the dip stand aren't adjustable. If they are, however, adjust them to a width that's as close to your body as possible, without touching your hips.

3. Use the foot steps provided to get up to the starting position. Place one hand on each of the dip stand arms, palms facing your body. It's best to grasp the bar with your thumb on one side and your fingers on the other so your hand can't slip off the bar.

4. Start with your arms completely straight, holding your body up unsupported. Cross your feet at your ankles and bend your knees so you don't touch the floor at the midpoint of the exercise.

Movement

5. Slowly bend your elbows and lower yourself down toward the floor until your elbows and shoulders are at the same level (your upper arm is parallel to the floor).

6. When you've reached this position, push on your hands to straighten your arms until your elbows are straight and you are back to the starting point.

Precautions

If you've ever dislocated your shoulder, or if you experience any shoulder pain while performing this exercise, do not continue. Try another triceps exercise in this chapter as an alternative.

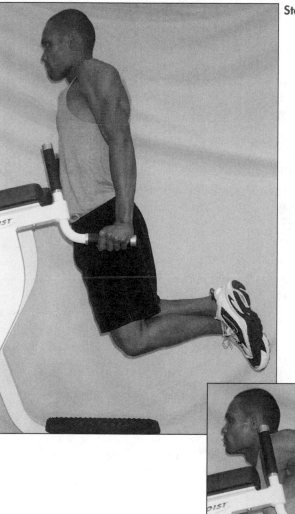

Starting/ending position.

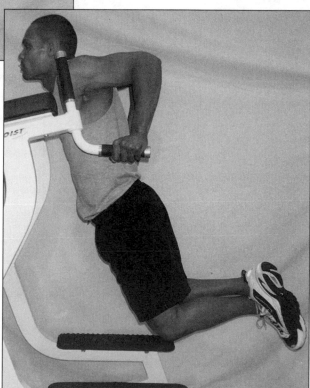

Midpoint position.

Assisted Dip

A few years ago, exercise machines such as the Gravitron (shown in the photos) were introduced, making it easier to do vertical dips. An assisted dip machine like this one uses a weight stack to counterbalance your body weight. The more weight you select, the less of your body weight you are lifting. This is the one time that adding weight to a machine actually makes the exercise easier. The concept is similar to that of a teeter-totter: If the weight you use is the same as or more than your body weight, the exercise is extremely easy. If you use less weight than your body weight, the exercise becomes more intense. Your ultimate goal should be to work your way up the weight stack until you aren't using any weight; instead, you're using your entire body weight as resistance.

Preparation

1. Typically, you can adjust the arms of the assisted dip machine to fit your body width. Move the arms of the machine to the position that is very close to your hips, without actually touching them.

2. Initially, trial and error will enable you to find the right weight for your current strength level. It's better to start with too much weight than too little (again, one of the rare occasions you'll hear this advice during strength training). Some machines have a chart that advises you on the proper weight to select for your current body weight. This is a good starting point. Be sure the selector pin is inserted all the way under the weight you choose.

3. Climb up onto the machine using the foot steps provided. If you are using a Gravitron machine, place your knees on the knee pad in the areas indicated. If you are using another brand of assisted dip machine, you may be standing on a plate rather than kneeling. Either way is fine.

4. Hold on to the machine's arms, with one hand on each side. Your palms should be facing toward you, and you should use a grip that places your thumb on one side of the bar and your fingers on the other side. Begin with your arms completely straight.

Movement

5. Slowly bend your arms and lower your body toward the floor. Stop when your elbows and shoulders are at the same height, or when your upper arms are parallel to the floor.

6. Push on your hands to straighten your arms, bringing you back to the starting position.

Precautions

◆ Many people who do this exercise for the first time end up bending at the waist to help lift their knees and feet. Be sure to keep your body straight: Bending at the waist cheats your arms from getting the most out of the exercise. Focus on keeping your hips pressed forward during the entire movement to avoid bending.

◆ If you've ever dislocated your shoulder, or if you experience any shoulder pain while performing this exercise, do not continue. Try another triceps exercise in this chapter as an alternative.

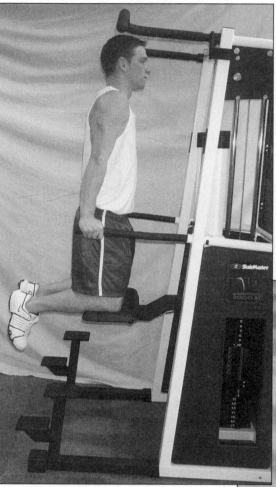

Starting/ending position.

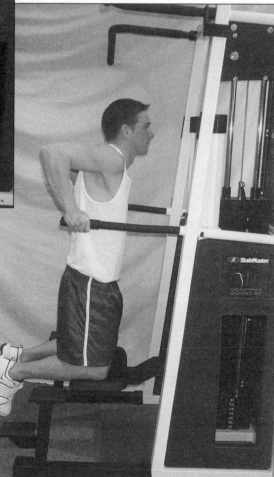

Midpoint position.

Dumbbell Kickback

The dumbbell kickback is a staple of triceps exercises. This exercise allows you to isolate each arm independently, giving each set of triceps muscles a lot of attention. In a normal standing position, straightening your elbow is as easy as just relaxing your arm; however, the kickback puts you in a position in which relaxing your arm bends the elbow, so you have to work to straighten it. I highly suggest you do this one in front of a mirror because you can keep an eye on proper form and the definition of your increasingly sculpted muscles.

Preparation

1. To work your left arm, place your right hand and knee on the exercise bench (or the edge of your bed). Hold the dumbbell in your left hand, palm facing your body. Your left foot should be on the floor.

2. Keep your back flat and your shoulders parallel to the floor. Don't "roll" your spine or lift your shoulders.

3. Lift your left elbow until your upper arm is parallel to the floor. Your elbow should be at about your side. If you get tired during the movement and your elbow drops from this position, the effectiveness of this exercise drops considerably. So keep that elbow high throughout the exercise.

Movement

4. Keeping your elbow, shoulder, and back still, extend your arm until it's completely straight and the dumbbell is back by your hips.

5. Slowly lower the dumbbell back to the starting point. Don't let the dumbbell "swing" back down or past the starting point.

6. After you complete a set on the left side, turn around, place your left hand and knee on the bench, hold the dumbbell in your right hand, and repeat the movement.

Precautions

If you have trouble keeping your elbow up in the proper position, spend some more time working on shoulder and back exercises—especially seated rows and dumbbell lifts—to strengthen your shoulder and back so you can get more out of the kickback.

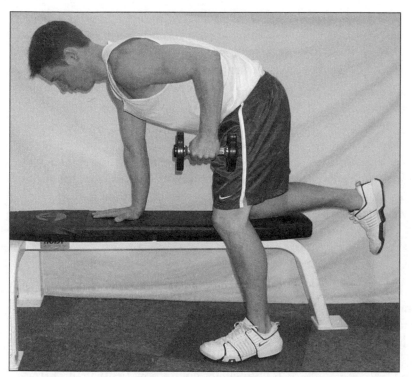

Starting/ending position.

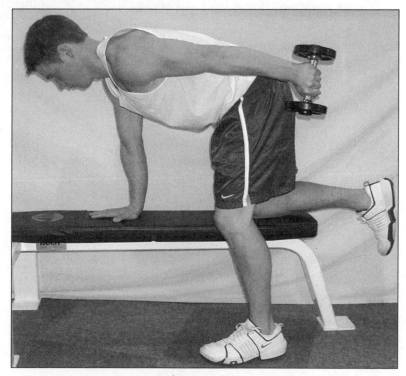

Midpoint position.

Tubing Kickback

Resistance tubing, which has gained much popularity in recent years, now challenges even the tried-and-true dumbbell kickback for bragging rights as a key sculpting exercise. In fact, it's even more effective. With a dumbbell, you work only about two thirds of the possible range of motion, meaning you get only about two thirds of the benefit. With tubing, you can adjust where the resistance starts so you get more out of each repetition. This yields faster body-sculpting results.

Preparation

1. Attach one end of your resistance tubing to a doorknob or a stable surface—something that will support the tubing even when you pull it.

2. To work your left arm, hold the free end of the tubing in your left hand, stand with your right foot slightly in front of your left, and place your right hand on your right knee for support. Bend forward slightly, but keep your back straight.

3. Bend your left arm, lifting your elbow at your side until your upper arm is parallel to the floor (your shoulder and elbow should be at the same height). Keep your left hand as close to your left shoulder as possible.

4. Back up until there is a little bit of stretch in the tubing. If you start the exercise with slack in the tubing, you lose a lot of its effectiveness. The farther you back up and stretch the tubing initially, the more intense this exercise will be.

Movement

5. Keeping your body, elbow, and shoulder still, extend your left arm, pulling the tubing out behind you. Straighten your arm as far as possible (completely straight is your goal).

6. Slowly let your elbow bend again, bringing your hand back to your shoulder. The tubing will tend to snap back quickly unless you control it (like a rubber band that has been stretched), so take it slow and easy to get the most out of the exercise.

7. Switch arms, and do a set on your right side.

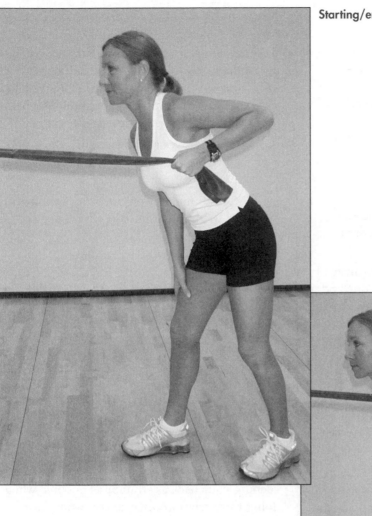

Starting/ending position.

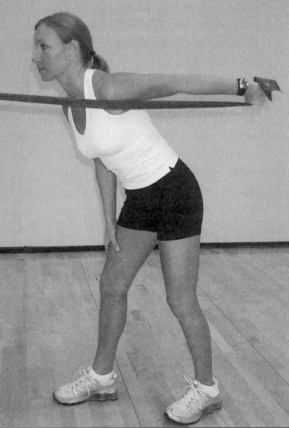

Midpoint position.

Overhead Press

The overhead press may seem a bit awkward at first, but after you get a few sets under your belt, you're sure to be comfortable with it. The advantage of this exercise is that the triceps start out in a slightly stretched position and must work even harder to overcome the resistance.

Preparation

1. Sit on an exercise bench or on the edge of a chair (be sure the chair has a short back).

2. Hold a dumbbell in one hand, but instead of holding on to the handle, cup one end of the dumbbell in your palm so you're holding the dumbbell the long way. Your thumb should be on one side of the handle, and your fingers should be on the other. See the photo for clarification.

3. To work your right arm, hold the dumbbell straight up slightly behind your head (don't hold it over your head, in case you drop it). Place your other hand on your knee for support.

4. Keep your back straight at all times.

Movement

5. Keeping your upper arm still, bend your elbow and lower the dumbbell behind your head. Try to keep your elbow pointed up at all times. Lower the dumbbell behind you as far as your elbow will bend.

6. Straighten your elbow and lift the dumbbell back up until your arm is completely straight again.

7. After doing a set on one side, switch arms and work the other side.

Precautions

Be sure there isn't anyone or anything behind you in case you accidentally drop a dumbbell. You may also want to use a spotter for this exercise, because the weight will be up near your head.

Variations

If the dumbbell becomes too heavy or big to safely hold in one hand, grip it with both hands to work both triceps at once. Concentrate on keeping your back as straight as possible when doing this variation because you won't have one hand on your knee for support. Your back has to do all the work to keep you straight.

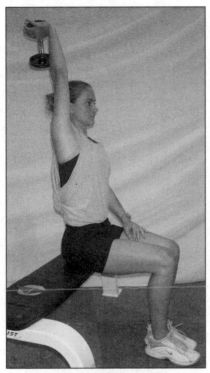
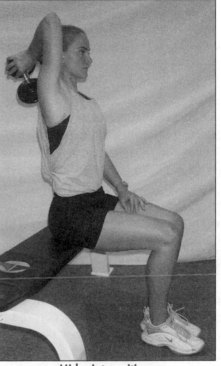

Starting/ending position.   Midpoint position.

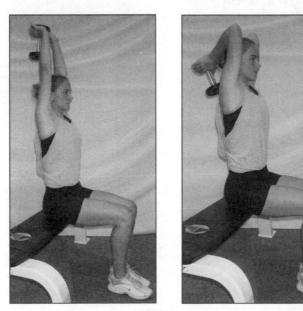

Variations.

Barbell French Curl

This exercise is one of the only effective methods of working the triceps with a barbell. Do not attempt it unless you have a reasonable amount of strength in your triceps already; this is an advanced exercise. The French curl is so effective because it stretches the triceps at the midway point, so the muscles have to work harder to overcome both this extra stretch and the weight of the barbell. Because it's more challenging, it's also highly effective for your sculpting goals.

Preparation

1. Lie on your back on an exercise bench or aerobics step. Place both feet flat on the ground for support and stability.
2. Using a shoulder-width grip, hold the barbell with your palms facing up. Keep your thumbs wrapped around the bar to prevent it from slipping out of your hands. Hold the barbell straight up over your chest and shoulders.

Movement

3. Keeping your elbows in the starting position and your upper arms perpendicular to the floor, slowly bend your elbows and lower the barbell toward your forehead. Don't let the bar touch your head or fall back behind your head.
4. When the bar is lowered within one inch of your forehead, use your triceps to straighten your arms, pushing the barbell back up to the starting point.

Precautions

This exercise has a nickname among those who do it frequently: the skull crusher. That's due to the dangers of performing this exercise without a spotter. If you don't have a spotter, try the dumbbell French curl or another triceps exercise outlined in this chapter.

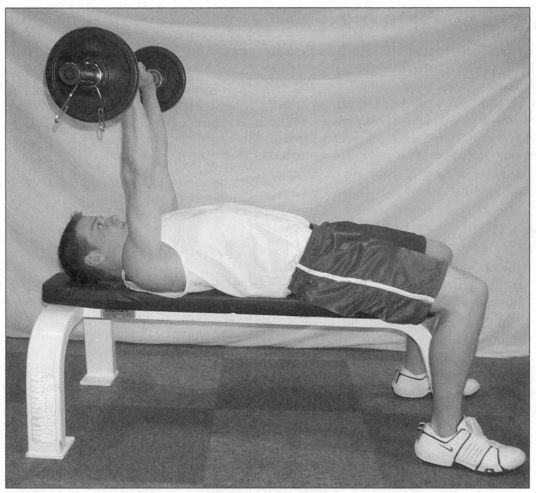

Starting/ending position.

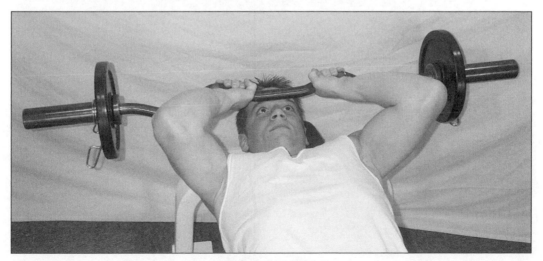

Midpoint position.

Dumbbell French Curl

Using dumbbells instead of a barbell for French curls allows you to isolate one arm at a time. It also means you don't need to have a spotter, so this is a good way to do French curls when you don't have a friend handy. This exercise really gives you a good stretched feeling at the midway point and offers great resistance through the full range of motion, making it excellent for sculpting the back of your arms.

Preparation

1. Lie on your back on an exercise bench or aerobics step. Place your feet flat on the floor for support and balance.
2. Hold a dumbbell in one hand. Keep your thumb wrapped around the handle to maintain a strong grip.
3. Hold the dumbbell up over your chest and shoulders. Place your other hand on your arm just below your elbow, using it to steady and support your lifting arm.

Movement

4. Bending your elbow, slowly lower the dumbbell until it's just beside your head at ear level. Your supporting hand should keep your elbow from moving.
5. Straighten your arm using your triceps, raising the dumbbell back to the starting position.
6. After doing a set on one side, switch arms and do another set.

Precautions

You don't need a spotter for this exercise because you can spot yourself with the supporting hand. If you have trouble completing a repetition, use the support hand to help push the dumbbell back up to the top position. Or just stop the exercise and use both hands to lower the dumbbell. If you feel more comfortable with a spotter, definitely feel free to use one.

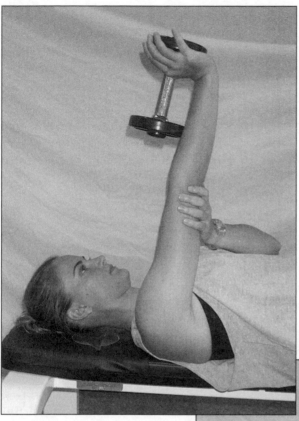

Starting/ending
position.

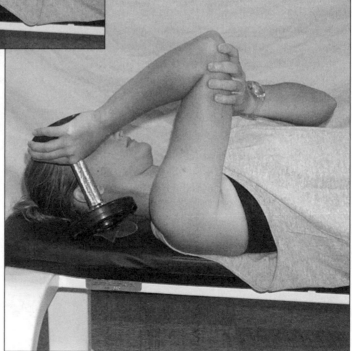

Midpoint position.

Triceps Press Machine

This form of the triceps press machine has become the norm for most equipment brands. It is basically the same exercise as the barbell French curl, except you are sitting instead of lying down. With an established range of motion and no chance of dropping a barbell, it's a safe and effective method of working the triceps.

Preparation

1. Adjust the height of the seat so that when you put your arms on the pad, your elbow and a large portion of your upper arms are touching the pad. If only your elbows are touching the pad, you are seated too high. If your elbows aren't touching the pad, you're seated too low.

2. Slide forward or back in the seat until your elbows line up with the pivot point of the machine. The pivot point is where the handles are attached to the axis of the machine; it's usually explained on the machine's instruction card or painted a different color than the machine. Line up your elbows with the pivot point so you are working *with* the machine, not against it.

3. You don't need to use the back support pad if you can maintain a straight seated position, but if it's more comfortable, adjust it so it just touches your back.

4. Place your feet flat on the floor in front of you.

5. Grasp the handles, one in each hand, and pivot the handle arm back toward you. It may feel a bit awkward at first, but that will pass when you get the hang of the exercise.

Movement

6. Keep your elbows in place, and push against the handles until your arms are completely straight.

7. Slowly bend your elbows back up to return the handles to the start position. This is the most intense part of the exercise because you really have to work your triceps to keep your elbows from rising up from the pad. You'll probably feel your triceps muscles "burn" with the effort.

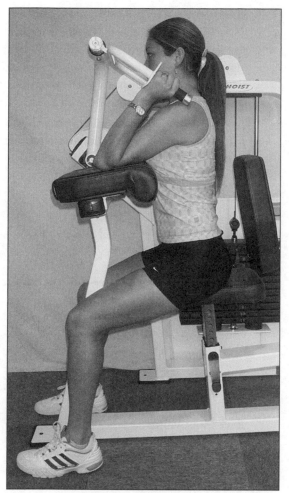

Starting/ending position.

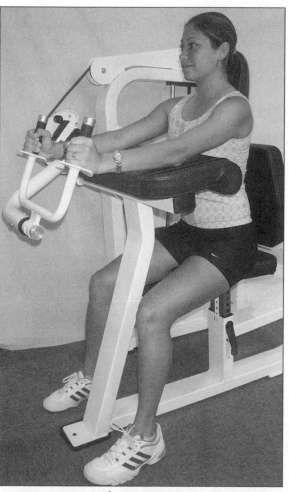

Midpoint position.

Cable Pushdown

Using a high-pulley machine, the cable pushdown simulates the motion of getting up from a chair, getting out of the swimming pool, or closing your suitcase when it's too full. The cable pushdown exercise provides a full range of motion, and you don't have to concentrate on balancing or holding on to a barbell, dumbbell, or tubing. Instead, you can relax your grip a bit and really focus your effort on working your triceps, without expending extra energy hanging on to a handle.

Preparation

1. Attach a straight handle or a triceps V-handle to the high-pulley cable. You can use many different types of handles for this exercise, but the straight or triceps V-handle supports the best form. Some bodybuilders like to use a handle made of rope, but that just makes your forearms work harder, which is not the focus of this exercise.

2. Grasp the handle, with one hand on each side of the cable, evenly spaced from the middle to prevent tilting. Use an overhand grip (palms facing down). Keep your grip relaxed, and focus on pushing down with the flat part of your palms.

3. Stand as close to the cable as possible without getting under it. If you find that the handle is swinging away from you during the exercise, you are too close; back up. Keep your feet apart, with one foot in front of the other for good balance.

4. Gripping the handle, bend your elbows so your hands come as close to your shoulders as possible. This is your starting position and is the highest point your hands will be positioned during the exercise.

Movement

5. Keep your elbows at your sides. Without swinging your body or leaning over the handle, push down with both arms until your elbows are straight.

6. Slowly let your elbows bend, and bring the handle back up to the starting position. Keep your elbows at your sides throughout this exercise. If your elbows start to move forward, don't raise your hands any higher.

Variations

You can do this exercise one arm at a time by using a single-handed attachment. This allows you to isolate each arm by itself and can help you to overcome strength imbalances between arms.

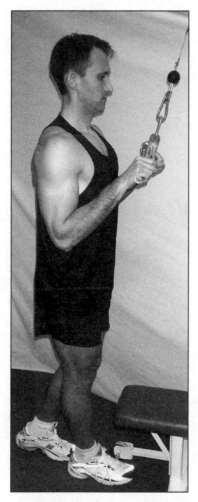

Starting/ending position.

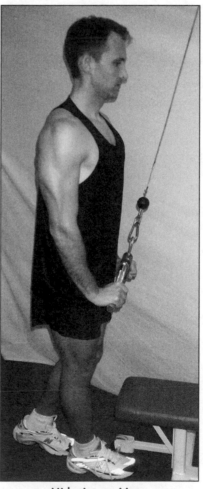

Midpoint position.

Tubing Pushdown

The tubing pushdown is almost exactly like the cable pushdown except that as you get closer to the midway point, the resistance increases as the tubing stretches. The triceps are strongest at full extension (elbows straight), so adding resistance near the midway point is a benefit that leads to more effective sculpting.

Preparation

1. Attach the tubing to the top of a doorway, or loop it over the top of a tall machine in the gym. Be sure each side is hanging down at an equal length, or you'll end up working one arm harder than the other.

2. Grasp one end of the tubing in each hand using an overhand grip (palms facing down).

3. Stand as close to the tubing as possible without getting underneath it, with your feet apart and one foot in front of the other.

4. Keeping your elbows at your sides, bend your arms so your hands are as close to your shoulders as possible.

5. The tubing should have some stretch in it at this point. If the tubing is too long, you may have to do this exercise kneeling on the floor (which is usually the case), or you can back up a little bit. I recommend kneeling instead of backing up. Backing up will cause you to work other muscles in addition to the triceps, which will weaken the effectiveness on just the triceps.

Movement

6. Keep your elbows at your sides while you press your hands down. Your goal is to get your arms completely straight.

7. Slowly let both hands return to their starting position near your shoulders.

Precautions

The tubing will be really stretched out, so be sure you slowly return it to the starting position. If you let your arms be yanked back up, you lose about half the benefit of this exercise.

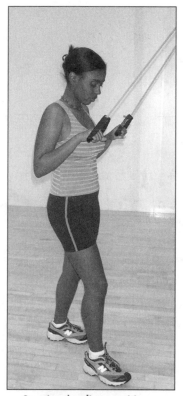

Starting/ending position—
standing.

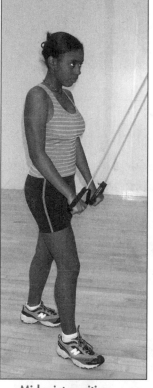

Midpoint position—
standing.

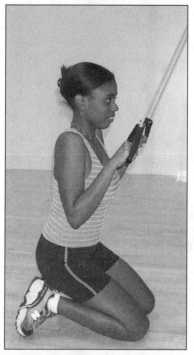

Starting/ending position—kneeling.

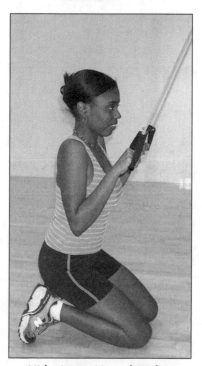

Midpoint position—kneeling.

In This Chapter

◆ Sculpting your backside through traditional floor exercises

◆ Proper use of specialized machines

◆ Using cable pulleys and resistance tubing to make your workout more challenging

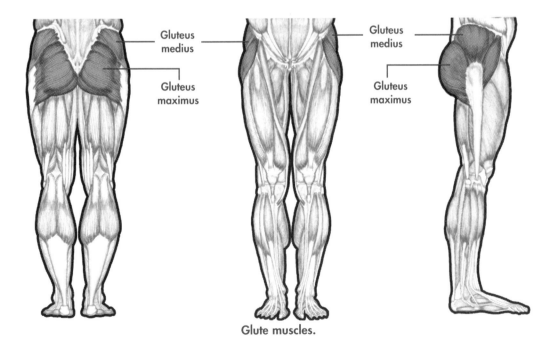

| | Gluteus medius | | Gluteus medius |
| Gluteus maximus | | Gluteus maximus |

Glute muscles.

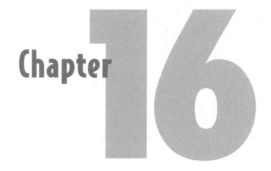

Chapter

Backside Basics

Men and women alike crave shapely glutes (a.k.a. butts). For women, glutes and the adjacent hip area are among the most common places to store excess fat; for men, this area is often simply ignored. But there are some definite advantages to strengthening your glute muscles, formally known as the gluteus medius and gluteus maximus. These are powerhouse muscles. They provide the drive that gets your legs moving. Because they are considered part of your core muscles, strong glutes provide a good foundation for sculpting your lower body. And of course, working your glutes is also the only way to get that tight, firm butt you've been day-dreaming about.

Horizontal Leg Lift

Made popular by Jane Fonda, leg lifts target and isolate the glute muscles without the use of any equipment. Although they're simple, leg lifts are highly effective, producing the signature muscle "burn" that lets you know you're doing it right. Many versions of the leg lift exist, but most accomplish the same goal. Included here are the exercises I recommend to clients as the most comfortable and effective.

Preparation

1. Lie on your side on the floor (it's more comfortable if you have an exercise mat or a carpeted surface). Position your bottom arm (the one on the floor) straight out over your head, and rest your head it. Do not prop yourself up on your elbow.

2. Bend your bottom leg (the one on the floor) so your knee is in front of your body and your foot is behind you. This will provide a solid foundation to keep you upright.

3. Your free hand (the top hand) should rest on your hip or waist. Don't place this hand on the floor because you will end up pushing against it instead of using your bottom leg's glutes for support.

4. Hold your upper leg completely straight, just off the ground. Relax your foot (it doesn't help to point your toe, like some people think).

Movement

5. Slowly lift your top leg into the air as far as you can.

6. Now lower your leg back to the ground, stopping just before you make contact. Don't let the lifting leg touch the ground or your lower leg.

7. When you complete a set on this leg, roll over and work the other leg.

Precautions

It may seem more comfortable, but don't prop your head up by resting your elbow on the ground and your head in your hand. This causes your spine to become misaligned, which will eventually cause neck pain.

It's easy to get in the habit of "throwing" your leg up and then "dropping" it back down. Be sure to concentrate on using your glutes during each repetition instead of letting momentum do the work. Overly fast movements and "bouncing" your leg can even cause pain or injury.

Variations

After a while, leg lifts will become pretty easy and repetitious. To increase the intensity, add ankle weights to your top leg. Start with a weight of about one to two pounds, and continue to increase the weight as the exercise becomes easier. You will definitely notice a one-pound increase.

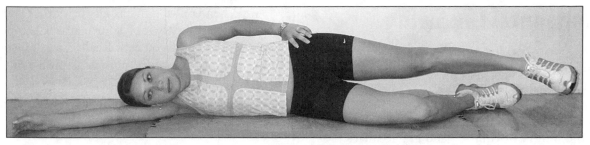

Starting/ending position.

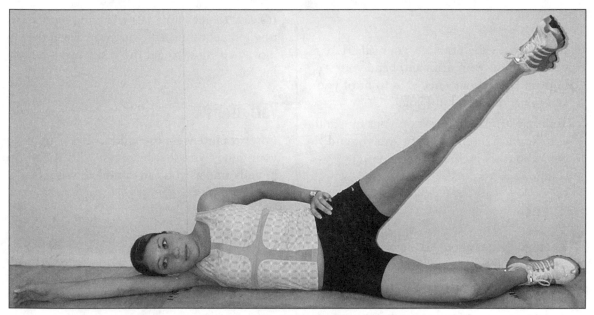

Midpoint position.

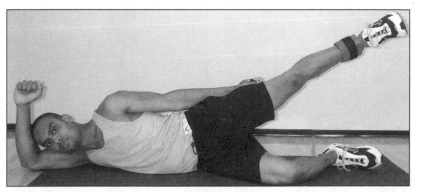

Variation.

Horizontal Leg Swing

The horizontal leg swing isn't something you'll find on the playground. This exercise works the glute muscles through their full range of movement unlike any of the other exercises in this chapter. The resistance you're working against is the weight of your leg and gravity that's trying to get you to put your leg back on the floor.

Preparation

1. Lie down on the floor, on your side. Lay your head on your arm, and bend your bottom leg so your knee is in front of you and your foot is behind you.

2. Your top arm should rest on your hip, and your top leg should be kept straight and held about six inches off the floor.

Movement

3. Keep your foot about six inches off the floor at all times; don't let it rest on the floor until you're done. Slowly "swing" your leg forward as far as you can without using momentum and without bending your knee.

4. When you've gone as far forward as you can, slowly "swing" your leg back behind you as far as you can. Really focus on contracting your butt muscles to push your leg back.

5. Repeat swinging from front to back, keeping your foot just off the floor.

Precautions

It's easy to get into a fast swinging motion, letting momentum carry you away. Keep the movement slow to get the results you're looking for.

Variations

For extra intensity, use ankle weights to make your glutes work harder. Start with one to two pounds, and as you can complete the repetitions, add more.

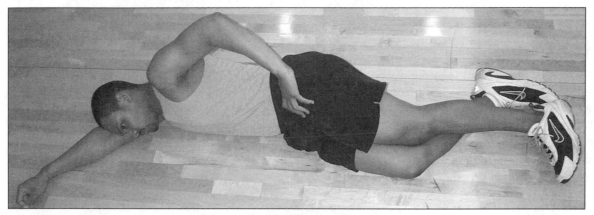

Starting/ending position.

Midpoint position—front.

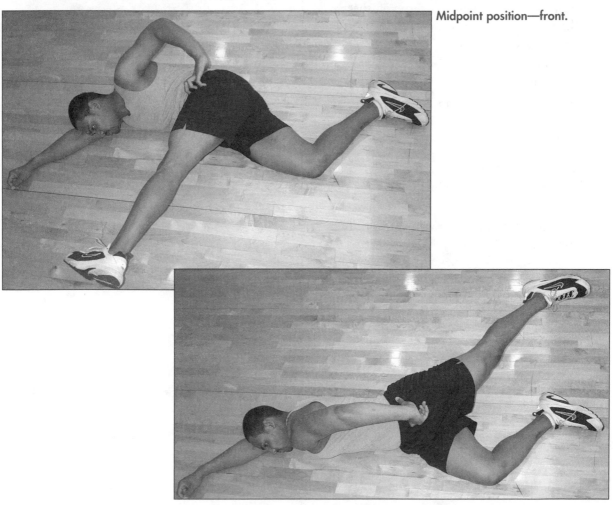

Midpoint position—back.

Donkey Kick

The donkey kick is one exercise that actually fulfills its name: The movement looks like a donkey kicking. Another type of leg lift, this movement focuses even more narrowly on your gluteus maximus (lower butt and "saddlebag" area). Besides the obvious sculpting benefits, this exercise helps you gain strength to do traditional leg lifts even more effectively.

Preparation

1. On an exercise mat or a carpeted surface, kneel on your hands and knees.
2. Place your hands directly under your shoulders and your knees directly under your hips.
3. Keep your back flat and your head down (don't look up, to the side, or back at your legs).

Movement

4. Choose which leg you want to work first. Keep your knee bent, and push the sole of your foot toward the ceiling. Move your leg back and up into the air in a smooth, slow, controlled movement (again, don't allow momentum to do the work).

5. Lower your leg back toward the ground without resting your knee and then repeat for more repetitions.
6. When you have finished with one leg, allow it to rest and gather strength for a few seconds before working the second leg, so you're sure it can fully support your weight.

Precautions

Be sure to keep your back as straight as possible while your leg is moving so you don't twist and injure your spine. Your hips may swivel a bit, but your back should remain still. Don't let momentum do the work.

Variations

For more intensity, add an ankle weight. Begin with a one- or two-pound weight, and move up as the set becomes easier.

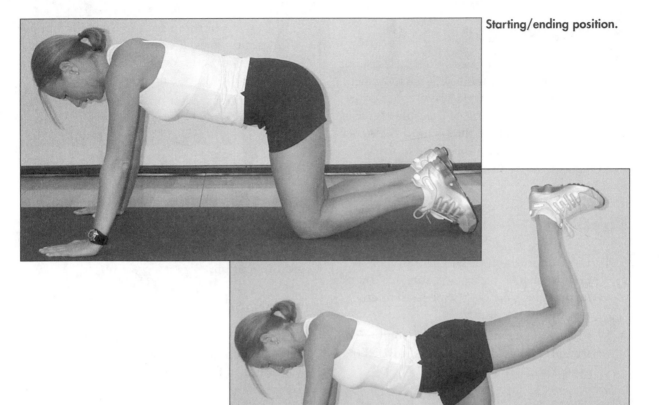

Starting/ending position.

Midpoint position.

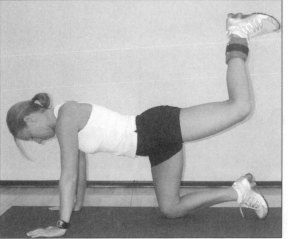

Variation.

Prone Extension

Prone extensions are similar to donkey kicks, but with a smaller range of motion. This movement is designed get the last little bit of contraction out of your glutes. It's one of the only exercises in which you pause at the midpoint of the movement so the muscle has more time to work. Although the movement is small, it yields big results.

Preparation

1. Lie face down on the floor on top of an exercise mat or a carpeted surface. You can lie on your arms with your head to one side for more comfort.

2. Place your feet together, with your legs straight and your toes pointed toward the ground.

Movement

3. Keeping one leg on the floor, lift the other leg as high as you can without lifting your hip off the ground. The idea is to make your glute muscles contract with a very small range of motion. Hold the leg up for a count of two seconds (one-one-thousand, two-one-thousand).

4. Lower your foot back to the floor, but just as it touches, lift it back up again. Don't rest between repetitions, and keep your repetitions close together and focused.

5. After doing a set on one leg, switch to the other side.

Precautions

Really focus on contracting your muscles with each repetition—don't go too fast. Hold each repetition for two seconds, lower your foot easily, and don't bounce your leg off the floor for the next repetition.

Variations

Add ankle weights for more intensity. Start with one to two pounds, and add more weight as you can handle a full set.

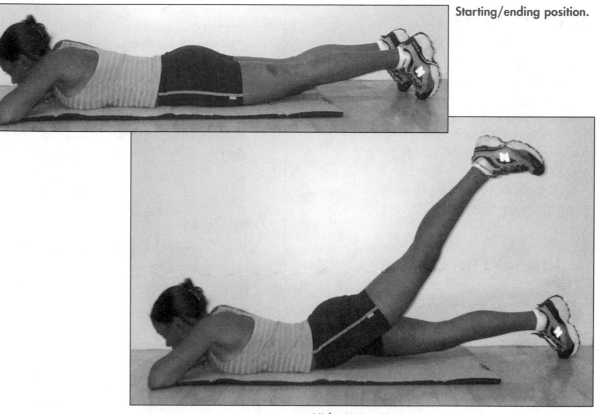

Starting/ending position.

Midpoint position.

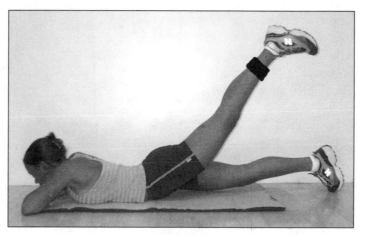

Variation.

Squat-and-Lift

The squat-and-lift exercise also uses your body weight for resistance. You work both glutes (left *and* right cheeks) during the squat and then isolate each side for a little more tightening. This is a multitasking exercise because you are combining the normal body squat (see Chapter 17) with a lateral leg lift for double the sculpting results.

Preparation

1. Stand with your feet shoulder width apart and your toes slightly turned out.
2. Hold your arms in front of you.
3. Keep your eyes focused directly in front of you (doing this in front of a mirror is best).

Movement

4. Slowly squat down by bending at the hips and knees (kind of like you're going to pick up something off the floor). Lower your body until your thighs are parallel to the floor. If you feel like you are going to tip over backward, lean forward a little more. As you squat, you should still be looking directly forward, not down or to the sides. Keep your back as flat as possible.
5. At the bottom of the squat, stand up by extending your knees and hips at the same time.

6. When you are back in the starting position, place your hands on your hips, shift all your body weight to one leg, and lift your other leg out to your side. Use your glutes to get your foot as high as possible (without kicking it up).
7. Place your foot back down, with your hands back out, squat again, and then lift up the other leg. Alternate leg lifts until you complete a set.

Precautions

If you find that you lift your heels during the squat or you cannot get down to parallel, stop where you feel comfortable or before you heels start to rise. With time, you will be able to go all the way down.

Variations

Add intensity with ankle weights on each leg. Use one- to two-pound weights to begin with, and increase the weight for more intensity as you can handle the repetitions. Always use the same weight on each leg.

Squat midpoint position.

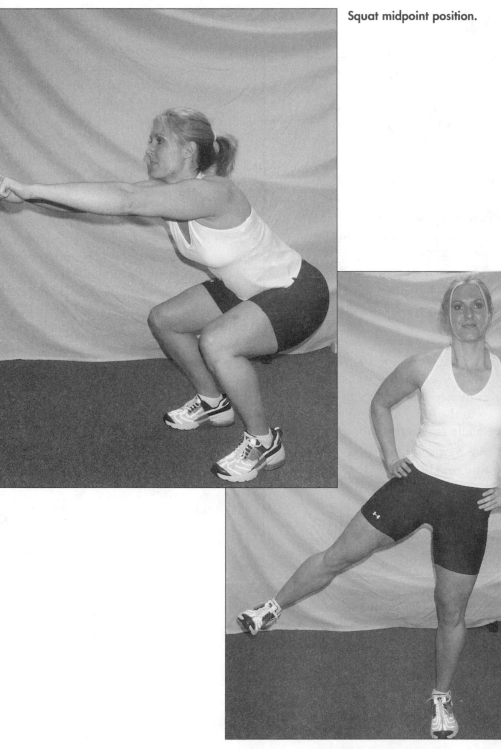

Lift midpoint position.

Side Lunge

The side lunge is a variation of the regular lunge that's covered in the next chapter. Whereas the regular lunge targets leg muscles such as the quads and hamstrings, the side lunge targets the glutes. Besides sculpting the glutes, the side lunge helps develop balance and stability.

Preparation

1. Find a hardwood or carpeted surface to work on. Be sure you are wearing good, solid athletic shoes.
2. Stand with your feet slightly apart, with your toes pointed slightly out. Place your hands on your hips.

Movement

3. Take a giant step out directly to one side. If you go to the left, keep your right foot in place while your left foot lunges.
4. When your foot lands, put all your weight on that foot, and bend your knee. Keep bending until your thigh is parallel to the floor. If you can't bend all the way to parallel, just go as far as is comfortable right now. Your other leg should remain straight.

5. Push on the bent leg to propel yourself back to the starting position. Don't push so hard that you'll fall to the other side, but push hard enough that you don't have to take another step to get back up (you don't want to drag your foot back to the starting point).
6. Repeat on the other side.

Precautions

The side lunge is a great sculpting exercise, but it can be hard on the knees if you don't take a big enough step or if you bend too deeply. When you bend down, don't allow your knee to jut out past your toes. Also, if your heel lifts from the ground, you didn't step out far enough. Be sure to take a big enough step.

Starting/ending position.

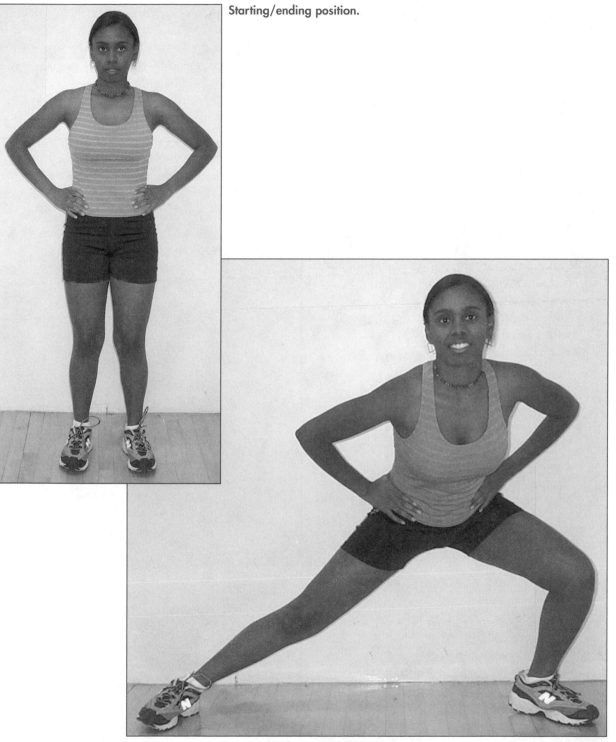

Midpoint position.

Glute Extension Machine

The glute extension machine mimics the donkey kick exercise, except it offers the opportunity to add resistance/weight to really make those glutes work. This is also a good alternative if you have knee problems and you find it uncomfortable to support your body weight on one knee during donkey kicks.

Preparation

1. Begin by adjusting a couple of the machine's features: the height of the pad that you'll rest your elbows on and the height of the pad you'll rest your chest on. Set both at a comfortable position that matches your body height. Don't hunch over the machine with pads that are too low.

2. Place one foot on the platform and one on the floor to support you. Place your platform foot directly in line with the leg being used (don't "reach" across the platform), flat in the middle of the platform so neither your toes nor your heels are hanging off.

3. Select the weight you want to use, and be sure the selector pin is pushed all the way in.

Movement

4. Push back with the foot on the platform as far as possible. It's rare that you will be able to completely straighten your leg because of the way the machines are designed.

5. Slowly lower the platform back to the starting position, but stop just before the weight stack comes to rest. This allows you to keep some pressure on the muscle, helping you to work it more effectively.

6. Complete a set on one leg and then switch to the other.

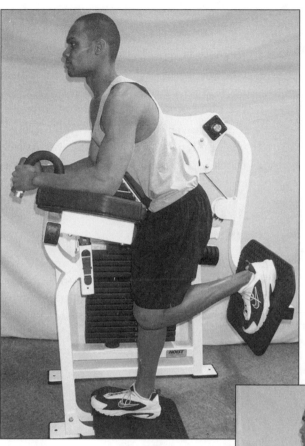

Starting/ending position.

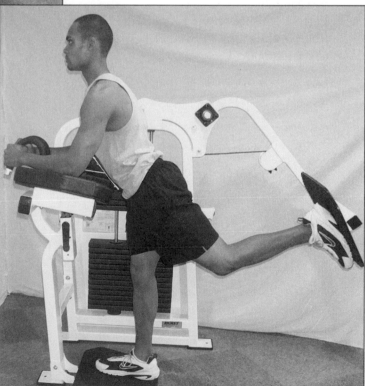

Midpoint position.

Hip Extension Machine

The hip extension machine mimics the movement of the prone extension, except you're standing up. The machine offers the ability to increase your resistance, working the glutes even harder. The machine also allows you to work both sets of glutes at the same time. While one leg is working to move the weight, the other leg is working to stabilize the body.

Preparation

1. The hip extension machine has one set of pads for you to rest your thighs against and one set of handles to hold on to. Standing as straight as possible, face the weight stack.
2. Select the weight you want to use, and be sure the selector pin is pushed all the way in.
3. Perform this exercise with one leg at a time, shifting all your weight to your stationary support leg.

Movement

4. Keeping your working leg as straight as possible, push back against the ankle pad. Push your leg back as far as possible, using the glute muscles to extend your hip.
5. Slowly lower the weight, bringing your leg back under you. Don't let the weight stack touch, or you will lose some of the intensity of the exercise.

Precautions

Although this exercise is relatively straightforward, there is still room for error. The most common mistake is to lean your upper body forward while you try to push your leg back. Be sure to keep your upper body straight, or you'll lose a lot of the exercise's effectiveness.

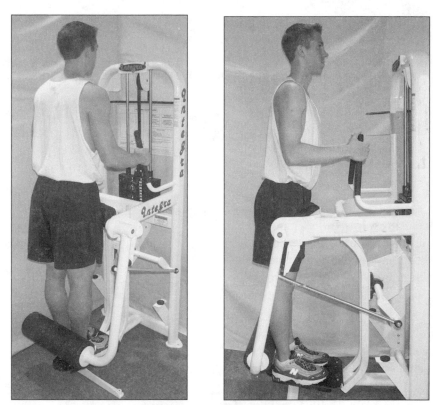

Starting/ending position.

Midpoint position.

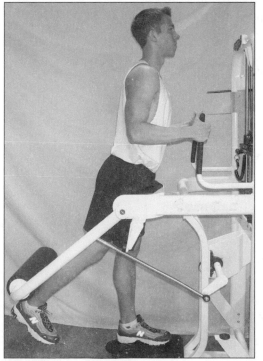

Cable Lateral Lift

The lateral lift can be done with either a low-pulley machine or resistance tubing. Both offer another way to add more resistance to the horizontal leg lift. When leg lifts become easy, add more resistance through a cable or tubing; it's the next level of glute sculpting.

Preparation

1. If you are using a low-pulley machine, attach the ankle strap to the cable and to your leg. If you are using resistance tubing, attach one end of the tubing to your ankle, and anchor the other end on something heavy.

2. Select the weight you are going to use from the stack, and be sure the selector pin is pushed all the way in. If you are using tubing, there should be a slight bit of stretch and resistance in the tubing at the starting point.

3. Stand so the leg you are going to work first (the one attached to the cable/tubing) is farthest away from the anchor (see photos for clarification).

4. Hold on to something stable with one hand for support. Place the other hand on your hip.

Movement

5. Keeping your body as straight as possible, lift the working leg directly out to your side as far as you can. Really concentrate on squeezing your glute muscles as you lift your leg. To maximize your range of motion—and results—shift your body weight over to your support leg.

6. Slowly bring your leg back under you and then repeat.

7. After doing a set on that leg, work the other leg.

Starting/ending position.

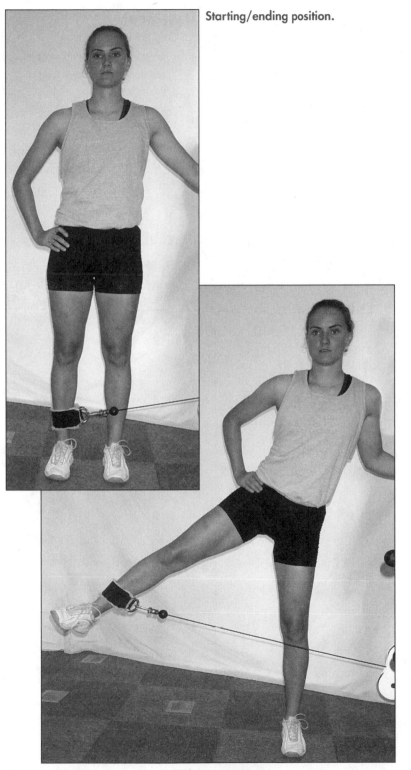

Midpoint position.

Cable Hip Extension

Hip extensions are also performed with either resistance tubing or a low-pulley. The low-pulley option tends to keep this exercise moving more smoothly. Tubing gets harder to work with as it stretches, and your glutes get weaker as you extend them (at the midway point of this exercise). Tubing can work, but a pulley system keeps the weight even throughout the motion so you can finish as strong as you start.

Preparation

1. Attach an ankle strap to the cable and to one leg.
2. Stand facing the weight stack. Choose the weight you want to use, and be sure the selector pin is pushed all the way in.
3. Hold on to the machine with both hands for support.
4. Step back just a little bit to put some resistance on the glutes at the starting point.
5. Shift your weight onto your support leg.

Movement

6. Keeping your leg straight, push it back as far as possible while really focusing on squeezing your glutes.
7. Slowly bring your leg back under you and then repeat for more reps.
8. When you finish with one leg, transfer the ankle strap to the other leg and complete another set.

Precautions

As with the hip extension machine, it may be tempting to lean forward to try to get more extension. However, leaning forward actually decreases the effectiveness of the exercise, so keep your body as straight as possible.

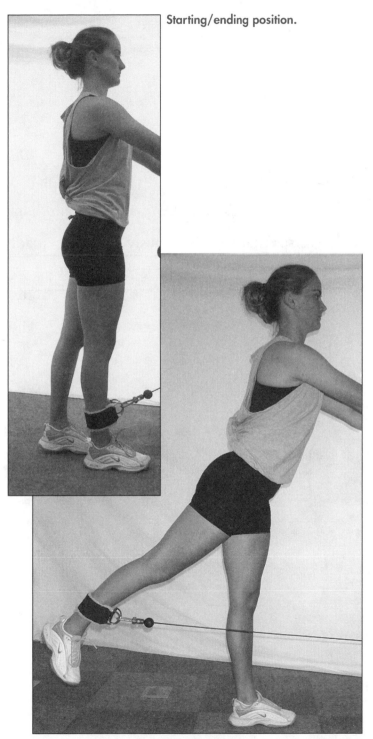

Starting/ending position.

Midpoint position.

In This Chapter

◆ Beginner through advanced squat exercises

◆ Exercises that isolate the quadriceps and hamstrings

◆ Exercises that simultaneously work the quadriceps and hamstrings

◆ Strengthening and sculpting the inner thigh muscles

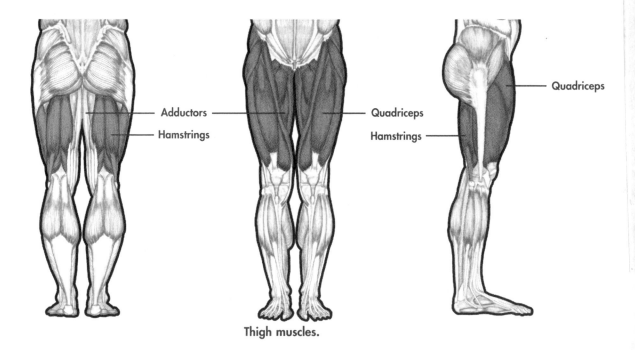

Adductors

Hamstrings

Quadriceps

Hamstrings

Quadriceps

Thigh muscles.

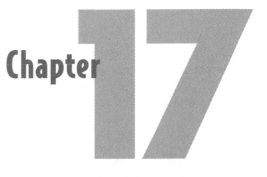

Chapter 17

The Thigh's the Limit

Your thighs consist of three muscle groups: the quadriceps, the hamstrings, and the adductor muscles. The quadriceps are the largest muscle group in your body, with four individual muscles that work together to extend, or straighten, your knee upon demand. The hamstrings are the opposing muscle group; located on the back of your legs, they work to bend, or flex, your knee. The adductors are the muscles of the inner thighs that work to squeeze your legs together, like when you ride a horse.

All three muscle groups should be trained as a group. Too often I see people working their quadriceps and ignoring their hamstrings and adductors—maybe because the quadriceps provide more visible results. But working the quads more than the hamstrings can cause imbalances that lead to hip and low back problems. Remember, all these muscles are connected to your pelvis and hip bones and so should be trained with equal enthusiasm.

Wall Squat

This chapter includes five squat exercises, and they are presented in order of difficulty. Squats are an important part of any body-sculpting program because they work all three thigh muscle groups and because the motion itself is so useful in everyday life. On the flip side, the squat has gotten some bad press as being dangerous for your knees. However, if it is performed correctly, the squat can improve knee stability. A squat will cause pain or stress to the knees only if performed incorrectly or if you already have knee problems.

The beginning squat exercise, the wall squat, incorporates a stability ball and a wall to provide support until your legs become comfortable with the movement. Try this exercise to determine whether deep bending will be okay with your knees.

Preparation

1. Standing against a wall, place a stability ball in the curve of your lower back, with the ball between you and the wall. Lean on the ball.

2. Place your feet about a foot in front of you, shoulder width apart, with your toes turned slightly out. Place your hands on your hips.

Movement

3. While keeping your back and torso as straight as possible, slowly bend your knees and hips and "squat" down.

4. Lower your body until your thighs are parallel to the floor and then push back up. To really focus on your thighs, think of pushing your feet into the floor. This concentrates the effort on your quadriceps.

Precautions

◆ As you squat, the ball will roll up toward your shoulders. The ball should never pass your shoulder blades. If it does, start with the ball placed a little lower on your back. Also, as the ball moves up and you move down, concentrate on keeping your back straight, and don't let your hips roll back under the ball. By keeping the ball between you and the wall, you'll also be working your core with this exercise.

◆ If you notice that your knees extend out past your toes at the midway point, place your feet a little farther out from the wall. This is where your knees risk injury during the exercise; you don't want them to bend too far. By placing your feet farther out from the wall, you can avoid this.

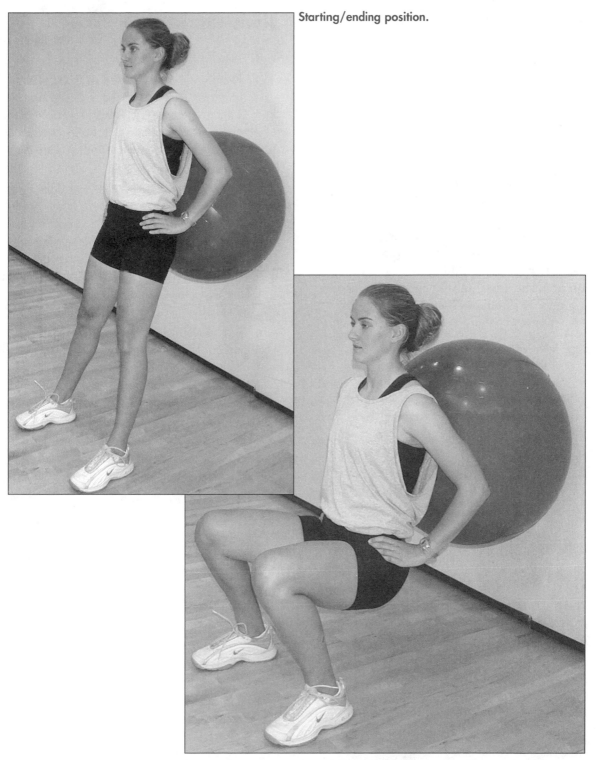

Starting/ending position.

Midpoint position.

Body Squat

The body squat is great for working on your thigh strength and your overall balance. The key to this exercise is getting low enough that your quadriceps and hamstrings both benefit. The body squat also helps you develop proper bending technique for use in everyday life.

The body squat is the technique you should use any time you bend to pick up something off the floor; do this instead of simply bending at the waist. As you squat, the hamstrings and quadriceps work together to control your descent (and keep you from plopping on the floor). On the way up, the quads work to straighten the knee, and the hamstrings assist the glutes in extending the hips.

Preparation

1. Stand with your feet placed slightly wider than shoulder width, with your toes turned out just a little bit. This should be a comfortable standing position; make adjustments to fit your normal stance.

2. Hold your arms straight out in front of you. They will help you balance during the lowest part of the squat.

Movement

3. Take a deep breath and hold it.

4. Keep your eyes focused in front of you. If you look down, your back will round; you want to keep it flat. This is a good exercise to watch in the mirror so you can see what you are doing without having to look down at your legs.

5. Bend your knees and hips, and lower yourself into the squat position. If you squat correctly, your hips will be behind you and your upper body will lean forward. You should feel balanced. Squat until your thighs are parallel to the floor (if your hips are lower than your knees, you've gone too far).

6. At the midway point, you should feel balanced. If you feel like you're going to fall backward, lean your upper body forward more. If you feel like you're going to fall forward, straighten your torso a bit.

7. Think about pushing your feet into the floor as you extend your knees and hips to stand back up to the starting position. Breathe out as you stand up.

Precautions

Never squat lower than when your thighs are parallel to the floor. Doing so can injure your knees.

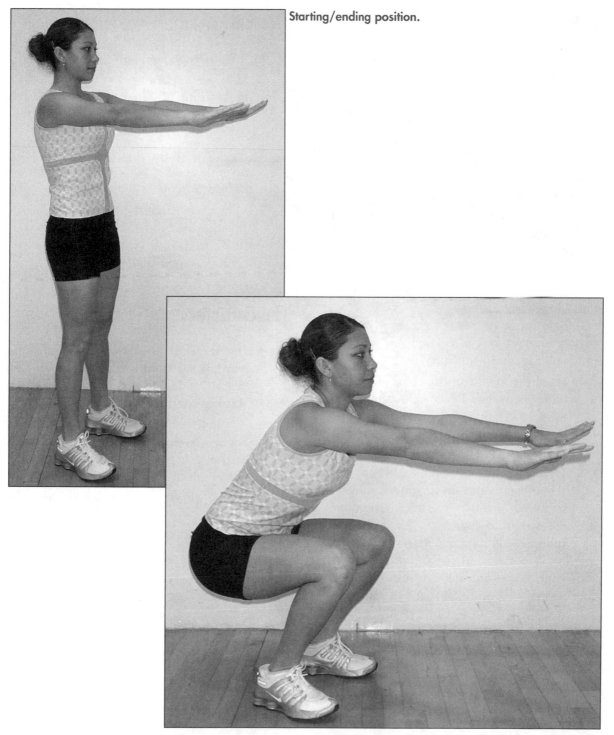

Starting/ending position.

Midpoint position.

Tubing Squat

Tubing is tailor made for the squat exercise, working your muscles harder at their greater points of strength. The weakest position of the squat is at the midway point, where the tubing is less stretched and not as difficult. As you stand up from the squat, the tubing stretches and the exercise increases in intensity, providing more benefit to your thighs. If you're a frequent traveler, bring along some tubing to keep up with your squats; it's easy to pack and very light. The tubing squat is definitely a "do-anywhere" exercise.

Preparation

1. Stand with your feet together. This is the only squat for which you stand with your feet together instead of apart.

2. Place the middle of the resistance tubing under both feet. Be sure the tubing is the same length on each side and it crosses under the middle of your feet (so it can't slip out).

3. Hold one end of the tubing in each hand. Bring your hands up to your shoulders, with your palms facing front and your elbows out to your sides. If it feels like the tubing is pulling your wrists and arms forward in this stretched-out position, wrap your elbows around in front of the tubing so it travels down the back of your arms instead of down in front of your arms. See the photo for clarification.

Movement

4. Inhale deeply and hold it.

5. Slowly squat until your thighs are parallel to the floor. You may feel a little less balanced than with the body squat because your feet are close together.

6. As you squat, keep your back as flat as possible and focus your eyes on something in front of you (such as a mirror).

7. When you reach the bottom of your squat, exhale and stand back up. As you stand, keep your back straight and concentrate on pushing through your feet.

Precautions

◆ If you feel like you're going to fall backward, lean forward with your upper body. If you feel like you're going to fall forward, straighten your torso a bit.

◆ This exercise really stretches the resistance tubing. Always do the tubing squat standing on a carpeted floor or exercise mat. A hard surface can damage the tubing, causing it to snap.

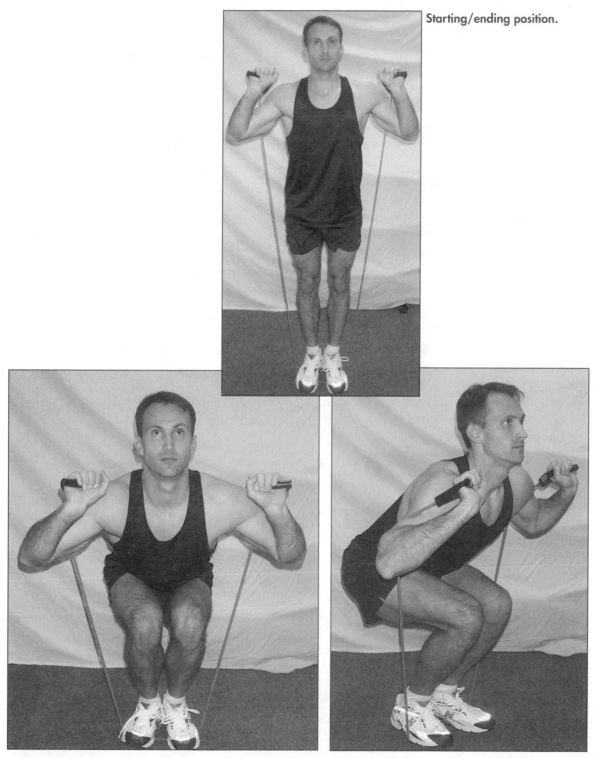

Starting/ending position.

Midpoint position.

Dumbbell Squat

Dumbbell squats really turn up the intensity by adding more weight to your squat. When tubing squats become too easy for your developing muscles, dumbbell squats step in to fill the void. They'll also prepare you for the even heavier weight of the next squat covered in this chapter: the barbell squat.

Like the body squat, dumbbell squats mimic the action of picking up objects off the floor (in this case, heavy objects). A good number of back injuries are caused by improper lifting technique in everyday life, so dumbbell squats teach you how to keep your body safe and strong.

Preparation

1. Stand with your feet about four to five inches apart, with your toes slightly turned out.

2. Hold a dumbbell in each hand, with your arms straight and your palms facing your thighs. The dumbbells are there simply to provide more weight—and, thus, more resistance—so all they have to do is hang. Keep your arms relaxed at your sides during the entire movement (but not so relaxed that you drop the dumbbells on your toes).

Movement

3. Inhale deeply and hold it.

4. Slowly bend down as if you were going to set the dumbbells on the ground beside your feet. As you squat, bend both your knees and your hips. Your hips should move out behind you, and your shoulders should lean forward. Really concentrate on keeping your back as straight as possible and your eyes forward (watch yourself in the mirror).

5. Squat until your thighs are parallel to the floor. The dumbbells may or may not touch the floor, depending upon how long your arms are.

6. Exhale as you stand back up. Concentrate on pushing your feet into the floor and raising your hips and shoulders at the same time.

Precautions

The most common mistake you can make with dumbbell squats is to lift your hips and butt first instead of standing up by lifting both the hips and shoulders at the same time. Lifting your hips first places extra stress on your lower back, potentially causing injury.

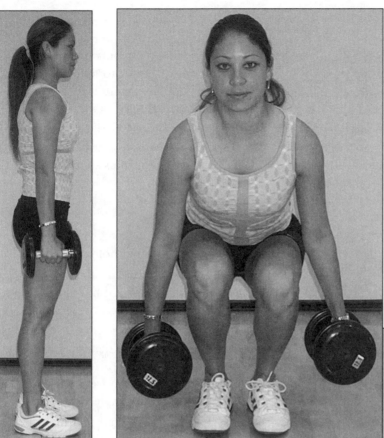

Starting/ending position.

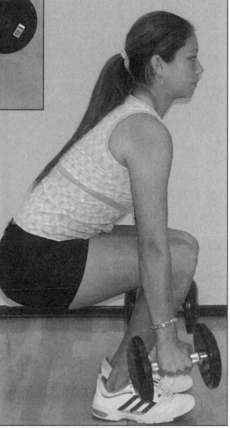

Midpoint position.

Barbell Squat

One of the three competitive power-lifting exercises, the barbell squat can be done with huge amounts of weight (I've actually seen guys with more than 1,000 pounds on the bar). Fortunately, you don't have to lift anywhere near that amount to get the results you are seeking. Most squat barbells weigh 45 pounds without added weight, which is plenty until you become comfortable with the exercise. The barbell squat is the most advanced of all the squat exercises and is one of the most difficult exercises in this entire book. With the addition of a bar across your back, safety is a major concern; this exercise should never be done without a spotter.

Preparation

1. The barbell squat should always be performed inside a squat cage. The squat cage has two upright bars that hold the barbell in place while you add any weight. With the help of a spotter, add weight to each side of the barbell at the same time (to keep it from tipping over), and use locking collars to secure the weights in place.

2. Adjust the catch bars of the squat cage so they are just below the level the barbell will reach at full squat. You can determine this level by doing a body squat and noting how low your shoulders get. Place the catch bars just below this point. These bars will allow you to set down the bar and weight if you have trouble completing a repetition.

3. With the barbell resting on the cage, duck under it and position the barbell so it rests across the top of your shoulders, just below your neck (see photo for clarification). If the bar feels uncomfortable, wrap it with a towel for extra padding.

4. Stand up with the barbell, take a small step back, and position your feet shoulder width apart, with your toes slightly turned out.

Movement

5. Inhale deeply and hold it.

6. Keeping your back as straight as possible, bend your knees and hips simultaneously and begin squatting.

7. As you squat, move your hips out behind you and your shoulders forward. Be sure to keep the barbell directly over your feet during the entire movement. Squat until your thighs are parallel to the floor.

8. Exhale and push your feet into the floor as you stand back up. As you stand, be sure to lift your hips and your shoulders at the same time, not one and then the other.

Precautions

Use a spotter and the catch bars! Spotters can help you maintain the correct position and help you with the weight when you get tired. The catch bars are even more important than the spotter: They prevent the bar from knocking you to the floor if you can't finish a repetition.

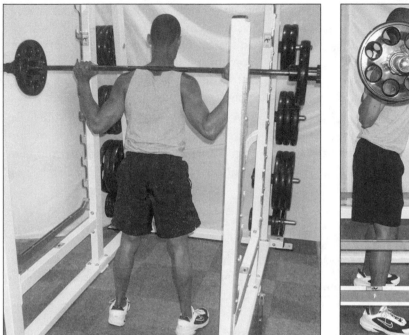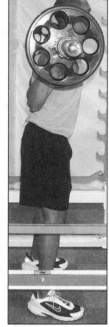

Starting/ending position.

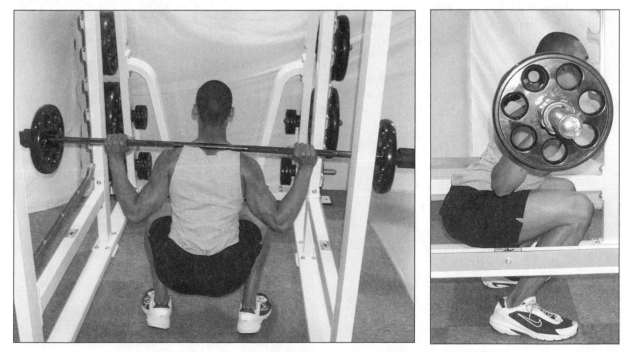

Midpoint position.

Lunge

The lunge really just consists of one big giant step, kind of like stepping over a big water puddle. A cool aspect of the lunge is that it makes both the hamstrings and the quadriceps work together, so you're killing two resistance-training birds with one stone. It's also an effective balance exercise, as you'll discover when you start practicing it.

Preparation

1. Stand with your feet a few inches apart and your hands on your hips.
2. You'll need an open space in front of you, so clear any obstructions.

Movement

3. Choose the foot you want to start with. Take a step that's about three or four times farther than you usually take. Imagine you are standing on narrow railroad tracks, with one foot on each rail. When you step out, stay on your rail and don't cross over to the other track. This will help you maintain balance.
4. As you step out, let both knees bend to absorb the impact. The back knee will move toward the floor but should never touch the floor. Stop when your front thigh is parallel to the floor.

5. Push on your front foot with a strong, fast movement to bring yourself back up to the starting position. Really harness some power to get back in one smooth movement. If your foot drags back, or if you need to take more than one step to get back, keep working on a stronger push.
6. Alternate left and right steps to complete your set.

Precautions

◆ At the midway point, your knee shouldn't be farther forward than your toes. If your knee passes your toes, your knee can become strained or injured.

◆ Your upper body is pretty much along for the ride with this one. Jerking back with your torso in an effort to get back to the starting position doesn't really help and could hurt your lower back. Concentrate on using leg power alone.

Variations

To add some intensity, hold a dumbbell in each hand. The extra resistance will make your thighs work even harder, for faster results.

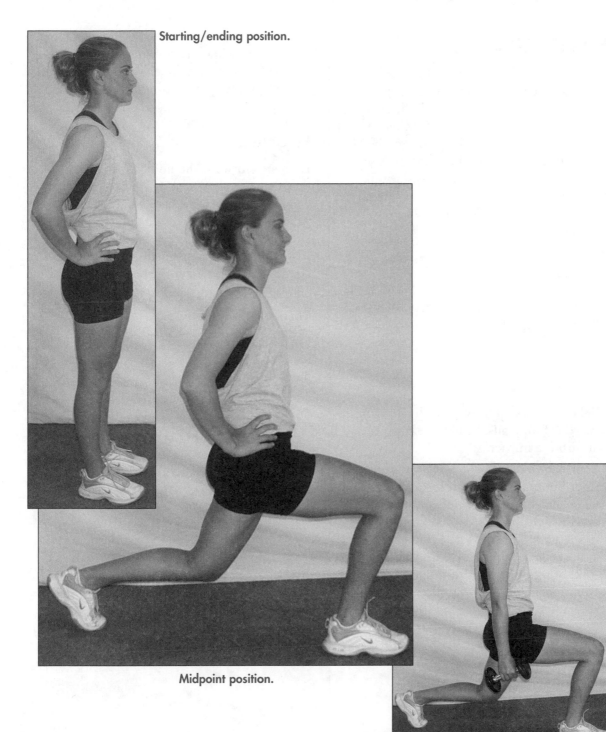

Starting/ending position.

Midpoint position.

Variation.

Walking Lunge

Although you may look slightly clownish doing the walking lunge, the results will be nothing to laugh at. Not only will you work the quadriceps and hamstrings with this exercise, but you'll also work the glutes, which help control the legs and maintain balance (three muscle groups in one!). You'll need a long hallway, sidewalk, or track for walking lunges—and remember, however far you go, you have to turn around and come back.

Preparation

1. Start by standing with your hands on your hips, feet slightly apart.

Movement

2. Take a giant step forward with one foot. As your foot lands, bend both knees to absorb the impact.

3. Your back knee should move toward the floor but not quite touch it (touching your knee to the floor puts most of your body weight on that one kneecap, which is not a good idea). When your knee almost touches, push up with your back foot, bringing it forward to meet your front foot. This whole motion resembles stepping over a puddle and getting to the other side.

4. Now step forward with your other foot (so you alternate working the left and right legs). Continue taking big lunging steps until you've completed your set.

Precautions

Each step forward should take you much farther than a normal step. If your step isn't far enough, your forward knee will pass your toes, which puts a lot of stress on your knee. Your knee should end up directly over your toes, not past them. Make adjustments to your steps, and after a while, you'll get the hang of it.

Variations

For added intensity, carry a dumbbell in each hand. Let your arms hang by your sides so the dumbbells don't swing.

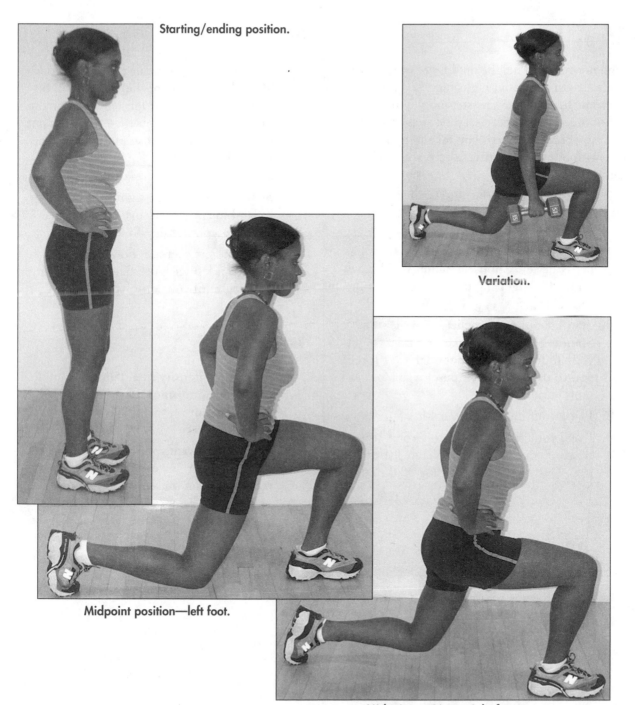

Starting/ending position.

Variation.

Midpoint position—left foot.

Midpoint position—right foot.

Step-Up

The normal step height on a flight of stairs or sidewalk curb is about eight inches. That's not very much, which is why stepping up on a curb is not much of an exercise. The step-up exercise supersizes the steps you take in everyday life, with enough repetitions to really work those thighs.

Preparation

1. Use any height of step you want, but bigger is better. Choose a height you'll have no problem getting up on or down from, though.

2. Stand about 6–12 inches from the step. Standing too close makes it harder to get your foot up; standing too far away forces you to use additional muscles and forward momentum.

3. Place your hands on your hips.

4. Place your right foot on top of the step. Be sure your foot is completely flat on the step. Don't let your heel hang off the edge.

Movement

5. Use the muscles in your right leg to push yourself up on top of the step. It will be tempting to use your left leg (the one on the ground) to help push yourself up, but that defeats the purpose of the exercise. Push with your right leg until you are standing straight on top of the step.

6. Step down with your right foot first. Try to land toe first to absorb the impact. Then let your left leg follow.

7. Continue the exercise, now stepping first with your left leg. Alternate starting with each leg until you complete the set.

Variations

◆ Add some intensity by holding a dumbbell in each hand for more resistance. Keep your arms down at your sides for better balance.

◆ If you really want to focus on one leg until it's burned out, instead of alternating legs, repeat steps on one side and then do a set on the other side.

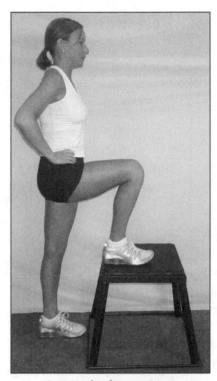
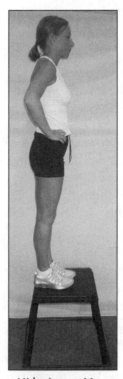

Starting/ending position.

Midpoint position.

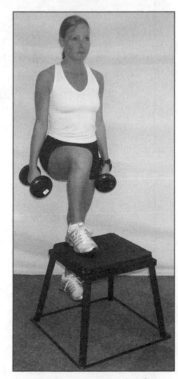
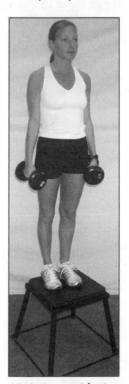

Variation—starting/ending
position.

Variation—midpoint
position.

Split Squat

The split squat is a combination of the lunge and the body squat. If you can lunge, you can do the split squat. The advantage of the split squat is that it makes the quadriceps in one leg work harder than the other, so you can focus your training a little more (it's like doing a squat on one leg). Training this small movement will enhance your ability to do the lunge and the walking lunge, and it is also great for working on your balance and coordination.

Preparation

1. Choose the leg you want to start with. You will do an entire set on one leg before switching to the other. Take a step that's about three to four times farther than you usually take. Imagine you are standing on narrow railroad tracks, with one foot on each rail. This will help you maintain your balance during the movement.
2. Place your hands on your hips.

Movement

3. Bend both knees so your back knee heads toward the floor and your front knee moves toward your toes. Keep your torso upright and straight; do not lean forward. Stop when your back knee is about an inch from the floor.
4. Push against the floor with your front foot, using the quadriceps in your front leg to do most of the work. At the same time, straighten by using your quadriceps and calf muscles.

Precautions

If during the downward movement your knees goes forward past your toes, you need to step a little farther out at the starting position. Letting your knee cross your toes puts too much strain on your knee.

Variations

You can add intensity by holding dumbbells in each hand to increase the resistance. Hold the dumbbells down at your sides.

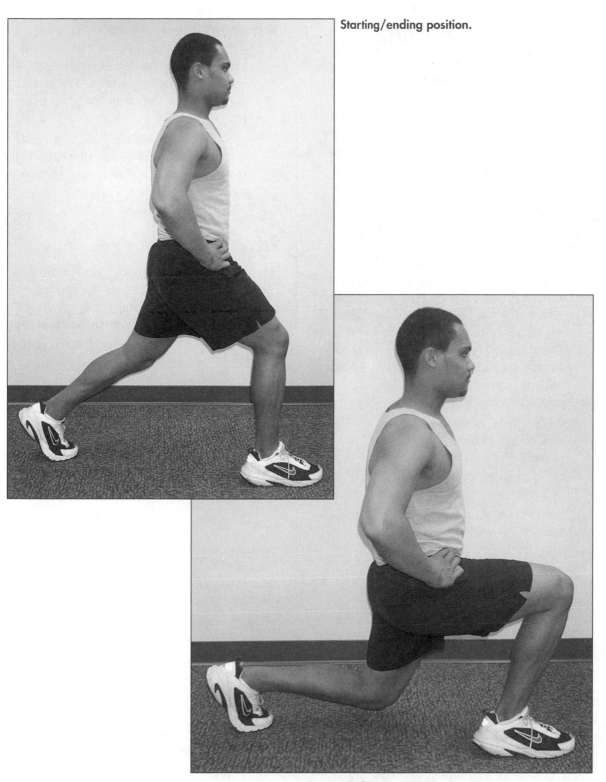

Starting/ending position.

Midpoint position.

Leg Extension Machine

The leg extension machine isolates the quadriceps, helping you create real definition. Almost all leg extension machines work exactly the same, so this description applies to virtually all manufacturers' machines. Because this exercise works only the quadriceps, be sure to also do either the lying leg curl or the seated leg curl to balance your workout.

Preparation

1. Sit down in the machine and adjust the seat back so your knees line up with the machine's pivot point. This point is always evident (or can be found on the machine's instruction card) and is usually at the edge of the seat. If your knees are too far forward, the beginning part of the exercise will strain your knees.

2. Place your feet behind the footpad. Adjust the height of the pad so it rests just above your feet, on your shins. You don't want it to push down on the top of your foot. Some machines adjust themselves, so you may not have to adjust it yourself.

3. Select your weight, and be sure the selector pin is pushed all the way in.

Movement

4. Hold on to the handles and straighten your legs as far as possible. The straighter your legs get, the more sculpting benefits you will see.

5. Slowly lower your legs back down to the starting position, but don't let the weight stack come to rest. Just before the weights touch, start another rep.

Precautions

This exercise should be done slowly and under control. If you go too fast by "kicking" the weight up and off your shins, the weight will be impossible to control and could cause injury. Be sure to maintain control and move slowly throughout the exercise.

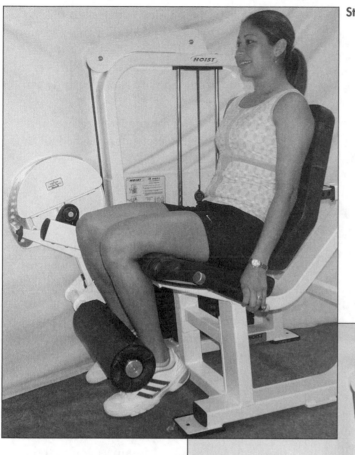

Starting/ending position.

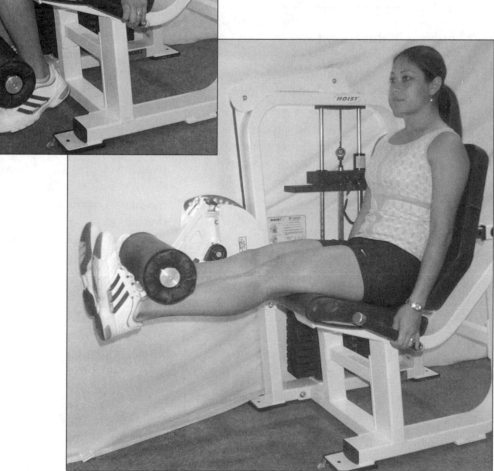

Midpoint position.

Lying Leg Curl Machine

The lying leg curl machine is designed to target the hamstring muscles in the back of your leg. The machine's position can be a bit awkward to get into and out of, but this exercise is highly effective for working this muscle group. Be sure to balance this exercise by doing leg extensions for the quad muscles in the front of your thighs.

Preparation

1. Determine the location of the knee pivot point on the machine. Most of the time, lying leg curl machines are designed so the pivot point is right at the edge of the padding. If this is what you see, stand at the end of the bench with your knees right against the padding, and lie down. Your kneecaps should hang off the end of the bench.

2. Some machines have pads for your elbows to rest on (top photo); others have a flat bench for you to lie down on, with handles underneath to hang on to (middle photo). Either way, lie all the way down, and put your elbows and hands in the proper position.

3. Your feet should be underneath the leg pad. Some machines adjust this pad automatically, but if not, adjust it so it is in contact with the back of your shins (your Achilles tendon) and is not pushing on your foot.

4. Select the weight you want to use, and be sure the selector pin is pushed all the way in.

Movement

5. Bend your knees and try to bring the foot pad all the way up to touch your butt. The farther you can "curl" your legs, the more you get out of the exercise.

6. Slowly let the bar back down until the weights almost touch. Then start another rep.

Variations

As the weights increase and the intensity rises, your hips will want to rise up as you pull on the bar. This is a normal body reaction to the mechanics of the exercise, but you can prevent this and focus on your hamstrings by pushing your hips down into the pad as you are curling your legs.

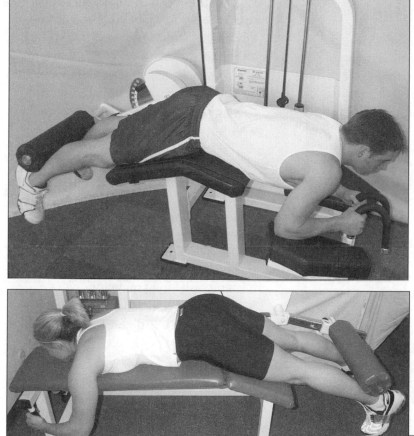

Starting/ending position.

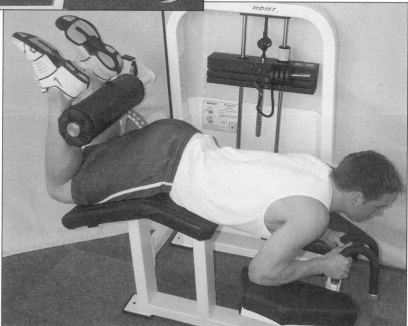

Midpoint position.

Seated Leg Curl Machine

Seated leg curl machines came on the market a few years ago and have since increased in popularity. Just like the lying leg curl, they target and isolate the hamstring muscles. A benefit of the seated leg curl machine is that it's easier to get into and out of, and you don't have to lie facedown on a bench to do it. The downside to the seated leg curl machine is that it offers a decreased range of motion compared to the lying leg curl machine, so it takes more work to get the same sculpting results.

Preparation

1. Sit on the machine and adjust the seat back so your knees line up with the machine's pivot point. The seat is usually quite short on these machines and may stop about halfway to your knees, so be sure to identify the proper pivot point.

2. Put your feet and legs on top of the leg pad. You may have to adjust the leg pad so it is in contact with your Achilles tendon and is not pushing on your foot.

3. Use the thigh pad to hold yourself in the seat; otherwise, when you push down on the leg pad, your knees will rise up and nothing will happen. Adjust the thigh pad until it's snug against the top of your legs.

4. Select the weight you want to use, and be sure the selector pin is pushed all the way in.

Movement

5. Hold on to the hand grips and bend your knees, pulling the leg pad down and under the seat. I tell my clients to try to kick themselves in the butt, although the machine will stop you before you do.

6. At the end of your pull, do an extra little squeeze to get a little bit farther. Every inch counts.

7. Slowly straighten your legs back out until the weights almost touch and then start another repetition.

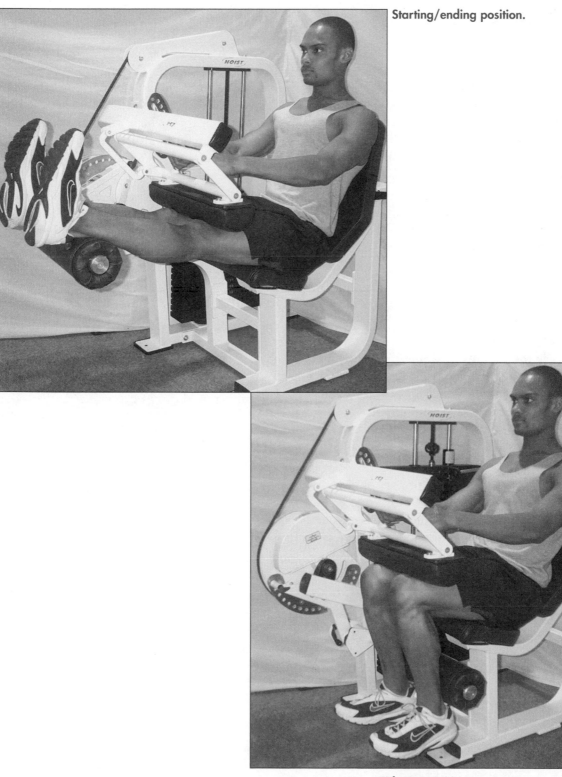

Starting/ending position.

Midpoint position.

Leg Press Machine

Want to work your quads, hamstrings, and glutes all at once? Then step right up to the leg press machine. A machine version of the squat, the leg press is all about moving even heavier weights by bending at both the knees and the hips. Unlike the squat, you don't have to balance because you are sitting in a machine.

The leg press machine mainly targets the quads and hamstrings, but the glutes also play an important role in getting you moving out of the midway point. If you don't like the idea of a barbell squat, but dumbbell squats aren't enough for you, the leg press provides a great alternative.

Preparation

1. Sit in the leg press machine and place your feet on the platform. Your feet should be spaced slightly wider than shoulder width, with your toes turned out just a bit (see the photo for clarification). Be sure to keep your feet completely on the platform; don't let them hang over the edge.

2. Adjust the seat forward or back until your knees are bent about 90°. Any greater than 90° will put too much strain on your knees; any less cheats you out of some of the benefits of this exercise.

3. Some machines allow you to adjust the angle of the back rest. This is strictly for your comfort.

4. Select the weight you want to use, and be sure the selector pin is pushed all the way in.

Movement

5. Push against the platform with both feet at the same time. When you push, put equal pressure on your heels and the balls of your feet. Don't allow the focus to be on your toes, which will make this a calf exercise. Push until your legs are almost completely straight, but don't let your knees lock.

6. Slowly bend your legs, letting the platform move back toward you. When the weights almost touch, start another repetition.

Precautions

It's nearly impossible to do this exercise wrong, but you can get hurt if you straighten your legs completely and lock your knees at the end. That puts unnecessary pressure on your kneecaps and can strain the joint capsules.

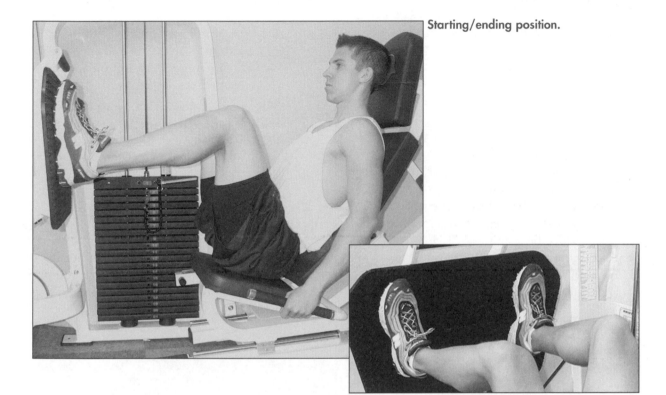

Starting/ending position.

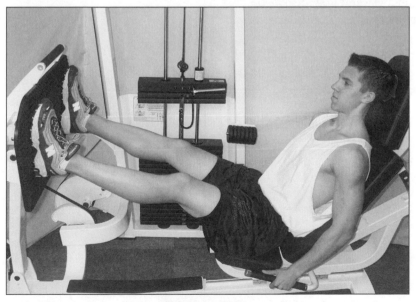

Midpoint position.

Thighmaster

Starting in the early 1980s, Suzanne Sommers gained renewed fame for hawking this nifty little gadget on TV. Although it has never been taken very seriously, the Thighmaster actually targets the same inner thigh muscles as the big, expensive equipment at the gym. I like the Thighmaster because it does such a good job of targeting muscles easily and conveniently. Unfortunately, working your inner thigh muscles alone—without cardiovascular activity and fat loss—won't get rid of the "inner thigh jiggle" caused by fat that covers the muscles. So for best results, be sure to do all your resistance training as part of a balanced body-sculpting plan that includes proper nutrition and cardiovascular activity.

Preparation

1. Sit on the edge of a chair, bench, or stability ball.
2. Put your feet together and place the Thighmaster between your legs. The "looped" ends of the Thighmaster should rest between your knees, with the pivot point directed toward the ground (see the photo for clarification). Hold the ends of the Thighmaster at your knees so it doesn't slide out.

Movement

3. Keep your feet together, and squeeze your knees together as close as possible. The Thighmaster will resist you and try to keep your knees apart.
4. When you've squeezed as far as possible, slowly let your knees spread apart until the Thighmaster isn't pushing against them anymore; then squeeze together again.

Variations

When you've completed a set working both thighs, you can also work one thigh at a time. Keep one knee still, and simply push in and out with the other leg.

Starting/ending position.

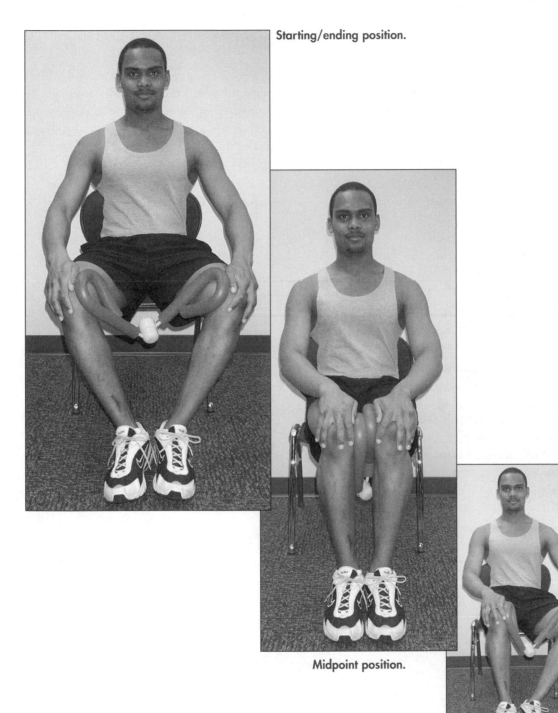

Midpoint position.

Variation.

Lateral Pull

Lateral pulls can be done using either a low-pulley cable or resistance tubing. Similar to the Thighmaster, lateral pulls target the inner thigh muscles (adductors) in an action that resembles kicking a soccer ball. This exercise provides a larger range of motion than the Thighmaster and thus gives better sculpting results.

Preparation

1. Choosing one ankle, attach it to the ankle strap from a low-pulley machine or to one end of a resistance tube.

2. Step away from the machine so the tubing or cable starts to give some resistance. Then take another step away.

3. Start this exercise standing on your support leg, with the leg attached to the tubing out to your side and up (see the photo for clarification). Place all your weight on your support leg, and lift your other leg out to your side as far as you can. It's not about how high you can lift your leg, but about how far away from your body you can get it.

4. Hold on to something for support, if you need it.

Movement

5. Pull your extended leg back toward your support leg and then across in front of your support leg as far as possible. As you do this, the tubing will be stretching—making it more intense—or the pulley weights will be rising.

6. Slowly move your leg away from your body to the starting position, and complete another repetition.

7. When you've finished with one side, switch the tubing or ankle strap to the other leg and work that side.

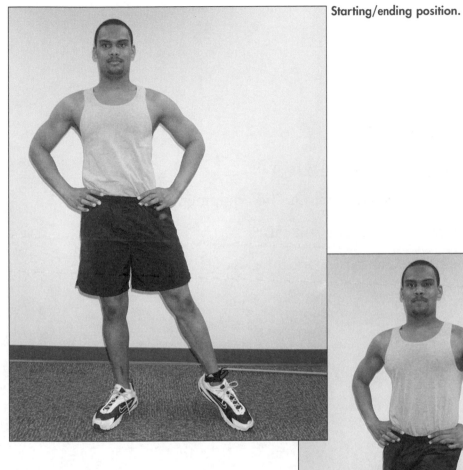

Starting/ending position.

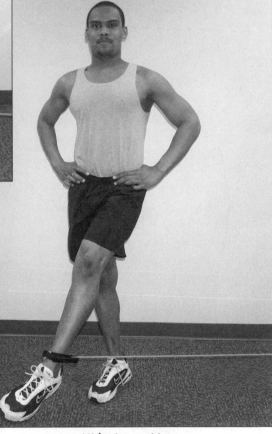

Midpoint position.

In This Chapter

◆ Using the calf muscles to walk

◆ Calf exercises that require no equipment

◆ Seated and standing calf raises

◆ Using machines to work the calves

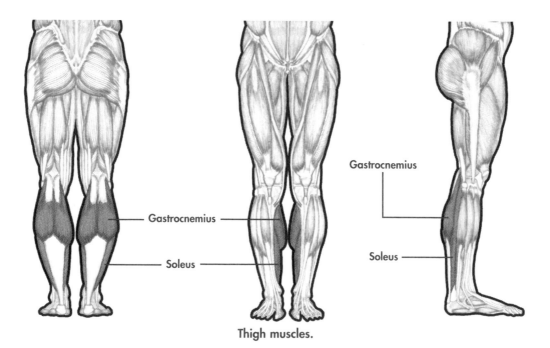

Gastrocnemius

Soleus

Gastrocnemius

Soleus

Thigh muscles.

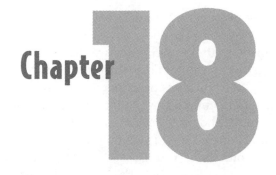

Chapter 18

Well-Cut Calves

The calf muscles are responsible for preventing you from lurching around like Frankenstein. Just try walking without bending your ankles or pushing off your toes—both movements that are controlled by the calves. But if they seem to be working fine, why sculpt them? For most people, the answer is as simple as this: Sculpted calves look good. Women know that high heels were made to highlight the calf muscles. For men, the calves are the only leg muscles completely visible when you wear shorts. Fortunately, calves are usually the easiest muscle group to sculpt, and the exercises are very easy to do (bonus!). There aren't as many exercises in this chapter because each exercise generally works the same muscles in the same way, so choose one or two you really like, and stick with them.

Standing Calf Raise

The standing calf raise can be done anytime, anywhere because you don't need any equipment. Standing calf raises are the most basic of all calf exercises. They are a staple of most people's leg workouts because they provide a great deal of definition by working both the gastrocnemius and the soleus muscles. Anytime you find yourself bored standing somewhere in line, do some calf raises. Everyone will think you're just trying to see over the head of the person in front of you.

Preparation

You can do calf raises standing flat on the floor or by standing on the edge of a step, curb, aerobics bench, or something similar. Standing on the edge of a step can be more effective because it allows you to drop your heels and stretch your calf muscles before you contract them. This provides you with a larger range of motion, which promotes greater sculpting results.

1. If you use a step, stand on the very edge of it, with just the balls of your feet and your toes on the step.
2. Let your heels drop toward the floor as far as possible.
3. Hold on to the wall or another object, to keep your balance.

Movement

4. Push up on the balls of your feet as high as possible. Be sure you use both legs and really get up. I tell my clients to pretend they are trying to reach something on the top shelf and to stretch as high as possible.
5. Slowly lower your heels back toward the floor, stretching your calves before another repetition.

Precautions

As you rise up and down, your feet will work themselves off the edge of the bench. Stop occasionally and reposition your feet.

Variations

For a really intense version of this exercise, use only one leg at a time. Crossing one foot behind the other puts all your body weight on one leg, making your calf muscles work twice as hard.

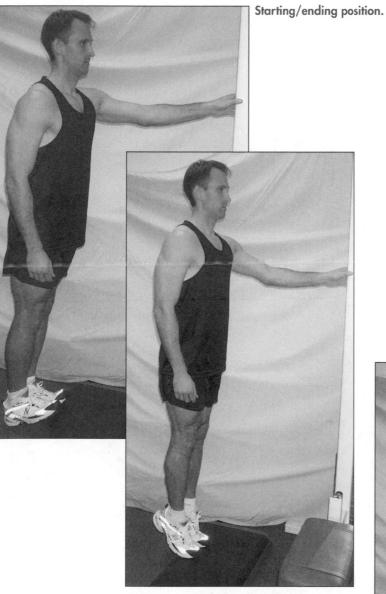

Starting/ending position.

Midpoint position.

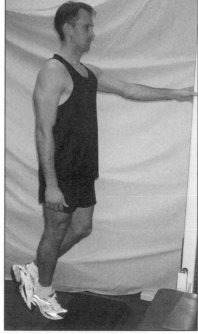

Variation.

Stability Ball Calf Raise

Unless you are a ballerina and can lift up onto your toes, the standing calf raise ends when all your weight is placed on the balls of your feet. The stability ball calf raise allows you to increase your range of motion even farther, and also utilizes your abdominal and lower back muscles to keep your body in a straightened position. So it's essentially two exercises in one.

Preparation

1. Kneel on the floor in front of a stability ball. Clasp your hands together and place your forearms on top of the ball. Lie down on the ball so your chest is on top of your arms (see the photo for clarification).

2. Straighten your legs behind you, placing your feet next to one another. Using your abdominals and lower back muscles, keep your body straight and rigid.

3. Rock back on your toes, pushing your heels as far away from you as you can.

Movement

4. Push forward, rocking up onto your toes. As you move forward, your body will roll across the top of the ball (if you roll over the other side of the ball, you've gone too far). Push up on your toes until you are as far as you can go. The goal is to extend the movement until you're on the tips of your toes.

5. Slowly rock backward, pushing your heels away from you again.

Variations

This is already an intense exercise, but if you crave even more, try isolating one leg at a time. Cross one foot behind the other, and let one set of calf muscles do all the work.

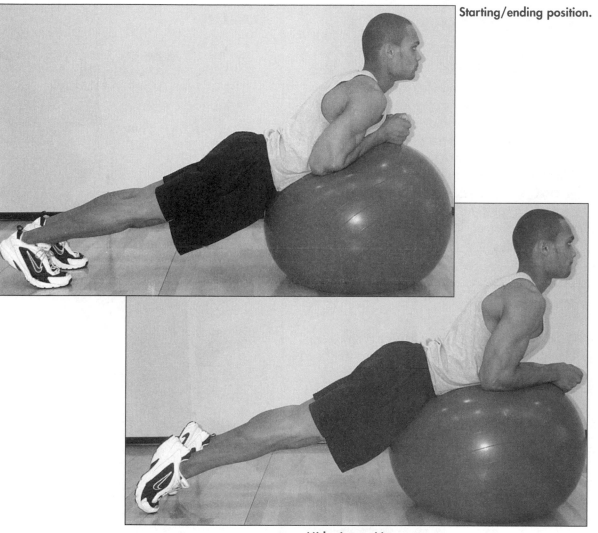

Starting/ending position.

Midpoint position.

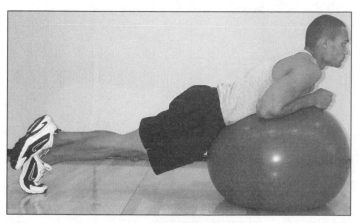

Variation.

Seated Calf Raise

The seated calf raise targets and isolates the soleus muscle in the calf. The soleus muscle is mainly an endurance muscle that's worked when you go for long walks, ride your bike, or climb stairs, so making it stronger will allow you to do more fat-burning cardio work. Because it's located under the gastrocnemius muscle, the soleus muscle is generally not as visible, so you won't see as much flexing—but don't let that fool you. Developing the soleus muscle will have a direct impact on endurance activities, helping you reach your sculpting goals on two fronts.

Preparation

1. Sit on the edge of a bench or chair. The bench's height should allow your thighs to rest parallel to the floor. A bench that's too high or too low will decrease the impact of this exercise. Sit with your feet together, flat on the floor.

2. If you'd like, place a weight plate or dumbbell on your knees for added resistance. You can perform the exercise without it, but the extra weight will provide better results.

Movement

3. Push up on the balls of your feet as high as you can. If you can make it up to the tips of your toes, you'll get even more out of this exercise.

4. Slowly lower your heels back to the floor.

Variations

Increase the intensity of this calf exercise by working one leg at a time. Straighten one leg in front of you, and let it rest while exercising your other calf.

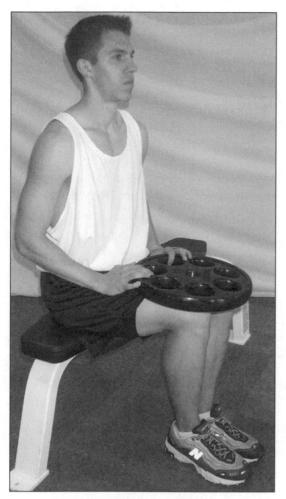

Starting/ending position.

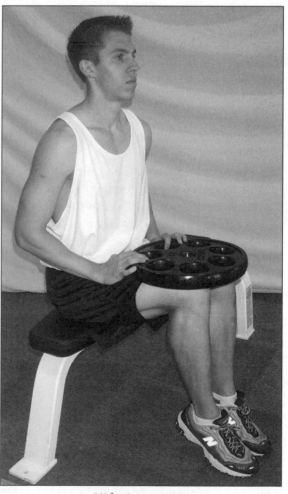

Midpoint position.

Calf Raise Machine

Old-style calf raise machines made you stand under a couple shoulder pads and lift the weight on your shoulders and back for calf resistance. Those machines ended up hurting people's shoulders more than they helped their calves, so a new style of calf raise machine has evolved. This model lets you sit and absorb the weight through your hips. Although it resembles a seated calf raise (because you are sitting down), it more accurately mimics a standing calf raise because your legs are held straight. This is a great exercise to try when regular calf raises become too easy.

Preparation

1. The calf raise machine has a pivot point around which the footplate moves. Using the instruction card on the machine, identify this point.

2. Place your feet on the footplate, letting your heels hang off the bottom edge. In most cases, only the balls of your feet and your toes will actually be on the footplate. Your heels should line up with the machine's pivot point.

3. Adjust the seat so your legs are almost completely straight. If you are able to hyperextend your knees (your knees bend backward a little bit when you straighten your legs), leave your legs slightly bent instead of completely straight. This will keep the knee joint from becoming injured.

4. Select the weight you want to use, and be sure the selector pin is pushed all the way in.

Movement

5. Push out on the footplate with the balls of your feet. The goal is to push your toes as far away from you as you can, getting your calf muscles to completely flex.

6. Slowly let your toes move back toward you, relaxing your calves.

Precautions

About the only way you can do this exercise wrong is if you turn it into a leg press. This happens if your seat is placed too close and your knees are bent instead of straight. If you see your knees moving during this exercise, move the seat back to make the most of your calf workout.

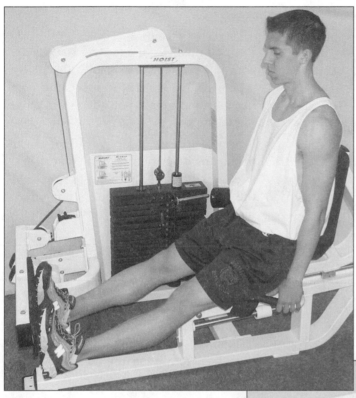

Starting/ending position.

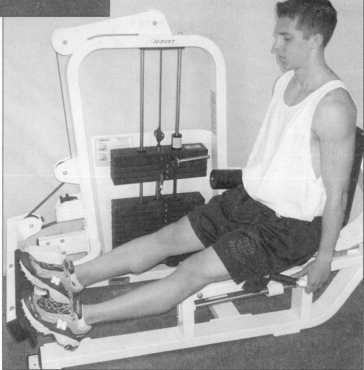

Midpoint position.

Seated Calf Raise Machine

Like the seated calf raise described earlier in this chapter, the seated calf raise machine also works the soleus muscle, but it adds more weight and a larger range of motion. Because of the added intensity, using the machine will lead to more sculpted calves.

Preparation

1. Place the weight you want to use on the machine.

2. Sit in the seat, place your feet on the footplate, and slide your knees under the knee pads. Adjust the knee pads so they are snug against your knees. Any space between your knees and the knee pad prevents you from doing this exercise correctly.

3. Most machines have handgrips on top of the knee pads for you to hang on to. You can hold on to these, or you can put your hands in your lap. If you do hold on to the handles, be sure you don't "pull" the knee pad up instead of using your calf muscles.

Movement

4. Push on the balls of your feet to raise your heels as high as possible. On the first repetition, the bar that supports the machine and weight you added will move out of the way.

5. Lower your heels as far as you can to get to the down position. When you can't stretch the calf any farther, push up on the balls of your feet again, raising your heels as far as you can to get to the up position.

6. Repeat lowering and raising your heels for a full set.

7. On the last repetition, when your heels are at the highest point, move the bar that supports the machine and extra weight back into place, and slowly lower your heels back to the starting point.

Precautions

Don't try to get out of the machine until the support bar is back in place. The support bar holds the extra weight you added. If you try to slide your knees out of the machine without using the support bar, you may injure your legs or damage the machine.

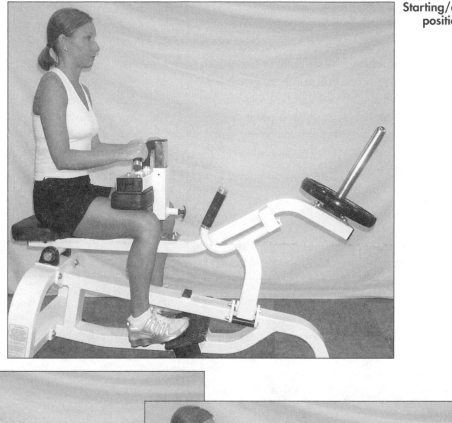

Starting/ending position.

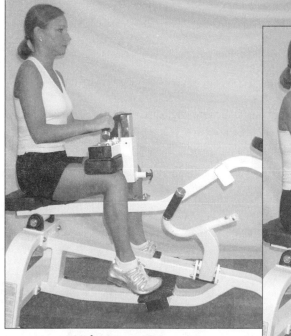

Midpoint position—up.

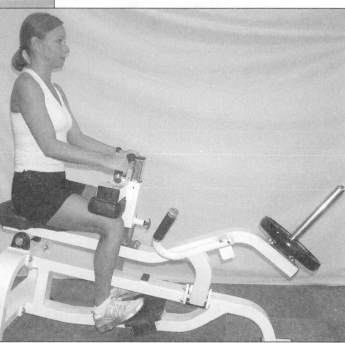

Midpoint position—down.

Tubing Calf Raise

The tubing calf raise is just like the standing calf raise, with the added resistance of the tubing to increase the body-sculpting results. This style of standing calf raise has to be done on the floor; you can't use a bench or step because the tubing will slip out from under your foot. You can make the tubing's extra resistance more intense by using heavier tubing.

Preparation

1. Place your resistance tubing under the balls of your feet, and stand with your feet together.
2. Hold the tubing as you would for a tubing squat—with one handle in each hand and your hands up by your shoulders—so the tubing is stretched to provide resistance.

Movement

3. Push up onto the balls of your feet as high as you can go. Really try to flex your calves and make yourself as tall as possible. As you push up, the tubing is stretched a little more, providing resistance to your calves in addition to your body weight.
4. Slowly lower your heels back to the floor, and repeat for more repetitions.

Precautions

Be sure the tubing stays under the balls of your feet and your toes. If it slips out while you have it stretched, it will pop up toward you like a rubber band.

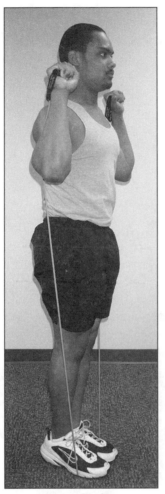

Starting/ending
position.

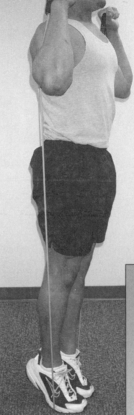

Midpoint
position.

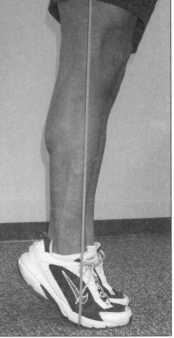

In This Chapter

- ◆ The pre-exercise check-up
- ◆ The best way to measure your progress
- ◆ Staying motivated for the long run
- ◆ How a personal trainer can help

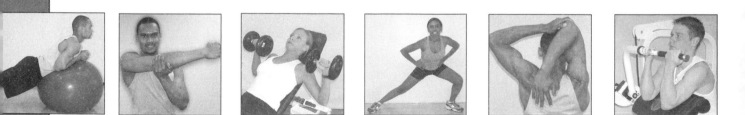

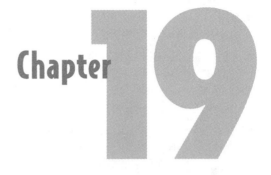

Chapter

19

Putting It Together

By now, your body-sculpting business plan should be written (figuratively speaking) and ready to implement. You should have an understanding of how proper nutrition will help you achieve your goals, which aerobic and resistance-training exercises you want to add to your regimen, and how stretching after exercise will keep your muscles and joints at their highest working capacity. Now all you need to do is put your plan into action.

This chapter addresses some final issues that may arise along your body-sculpting quest, including the most effective way to measure your progress and tips for staying motivated for the long run.

Before You Get Started

Before you begin any fitness plan, I recommend that you share your goals, and how you plan to accomplish them, with your physician. It's always a good idea to obtain medical clearance before you start a new exercise program, just to make sure that there isn't anything that might interfere or prevent you from reaching your goals as you have defined them.

Most physicians will ask you the following seven questions. A positive "yes" answer to any one of them may indicate that you should have a full physical and exercise stress test before beginning an exercise program.

- ◆ Have you ever been diagnosed with heart trouble?
- ◆ Do you frequently have pains in your heart or chest?

◆ Do you often feel faint or have spells of severe dizziness?

◆ Has a doctor ever said that your blood pressure was too high?

◆ Has your doctor ever told you that you have a bone or joint problem, such as arthritis, that has been aggravated by exercise or that might be made worse with exercise?

◆ Is there any other possible physical reason why you should not follow an activity program, even if you wanted to?

◆ Are you over age 65 and not accustomed to vigorous exercise?

Measuring Your Progress

It's all well and good to establish your goals and start following a body-sculpting plan—but how in the world will you know if you're making progress?

You may be tempted to rely on the scale alone to track your results. However, there are several ways to measure your progress as you work through your program, and the scale is usually not the best of them. That's because the number that shows up on the scale is a measurement that includes both your fat and lean weight (your muscles, bones, and water), without a breakdown of how much of either you have. Instead, you need to concentrate on changing your *body composition*—the percentage of fat in your body compared to the percentage of lean muscle. Quite often, my clients reach their body-sculpting goals and actually gain weight or maintain their current weight. If you stick with your body-sculpting program, your body composition will change for the better, no matter what the scale says.

Trainer Talk _____

Your **body composition** is the percentage of fat in your body compared to the percentage of lean muscle. Instead of focusing on your weight, measure your body-sculpting goals by analyzing your body composition.

For instance, if you start your program at 135 pounds, and you lose 4 pounds of fat during the first month but also gain 2 pounds of muscle, the scale will show that you have lost only 2 pounds (– 4 pounds of fat + 2 pounds of muscle). Two pounds may not feel like much, but you've also changed your body composition for the better, which means lost inches and a tighter physique. It's okay to gain lean weight and lose fat weight at the same time. And fear not: You will never gain as much lean weight as you lose in fat weight. Eventually, you will reach a point at which your gains in lean weight come more slowly, and you'll drop the fat pounds more quickly.

Fortunately, you can test and measure your body composition as you go. Your local fitness center should be able to help you with any number of body fat tests, including skinfold pinches that measure your body fat with calipers, water tanks in which you are submerged to determine body composition, and bioelectrical impedance instruments that measure your body fat via electricity (don't worry—you won't be shocked). I highly recommend that you measure this percentage before you even begin your program, to provide a benchmark for your progress. Of the methods available, I suggest using the skinfold calipers. It's easier than the underwater weighing and more accurate than the electrical method.

Over the course of your training, remeasure your body composition every three months or so (more frequently won't show your progress as well). All these tests measure your body fat percentage—obviously, you are seeking to lower this number as you go, which will indicate that you've reduced body fat and increased lean muscle.

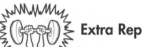

Extra Rep _____ To measure your progress, don't just use the scale. Get a body fat measurement at your local fitness center, and retest every three months.

Another way of checking your progress is very low-tech: Look in the mirror. During the first few weeks, you may not see a great deal of change, but this is because your body is changing from the inside out. Your muscles are becoming denser, and you're losing body fat. However, after you've been training approximately six to eight weeks, you will start seeing a noticeable difference in the way your body looks.

Regardless of how you look, you will notice one change almost immediately: how you feel. Your muscles will begin developing from your first workout, and you'll feel stronger, more energized, and lighter as you move. These changes can't be quantified with numbers, but you will recognize your progress by your increased energy level and reduced fatigue. This is what body sculpting is all about.

Extra Rep _____ You can also measure your progress by the way your body responds to your resistance training. As you continue your training, your muscles become stronger, and you'll need to add more weight to keep resistance training a challenge.

Finally, as you increase the weights you use in your exercises, you can't help but recognize that you are making progress. Your muscles didn't get stronger just by chance. Hard work made it happen, and now you can reap the rewards.

Staying Motivated

Maintaining the excitement and motivation you have at the beginning of your program can be a challenge. And inevitably, there will be times when you aren't motivated to keep up with your workouts. That's okay. You need to recognize that sometimes life's challenges get in the way, and something has to give. The key to temporary setbacks is this: Remember that you can always jump back into your program. As your body-sculpting program becomes part of your daily life, you won't be so quick to toss it aside when time gets short. It will become as natural as any of your other daily obligations, such as taking time to walk the dog or clean the house. Although it may seem difficult to imagine right now, there will come a time when you have difficulty skipping a workout. Exercise will become a part of your life that is always positive, always beneficial, and always just for you.

If your motivation wanes, go back to your journal and reread your daily goals—what you want to accomplish each day. Refer to this journal all the time, not just until you get the hang of exercising, but as a constant reminder of your original goals. These goals may change—and actually should change—as you go along. Your motivation will increase as you meet one goal and set the next. Above all else, remember that you can reach each of your goals with patience and hard work. The body is an instrument that can be molded into whatever you want it to be, as long as you keep working with it.

No Pain—Just Gain

Even if you miss a few days or even a few weeks of your workout because of life's inevitable challenges, don't give up. You can go back to your body-sculpting routine at any time.

Working With a Trainer

From time to time, you should meet with a professional personal trainer to give your program a boost. Even I, as a personal trainer, use other trainers and coaches to give me a kick in the pants and help me push myself to new levels. A personal trainer can help you to measure your progress, assist you in evaluating whether you are doing exercises correctly, and provide you with another means of motivation. I always want to give my trainer or coach a positive report when I see him or her; it pushes me to reach new goals and keep working harder.

You don't have to work with a trainer all the time. Once every few weeks or once a month for a program checkup is fine. You can find a professional personal trainer by calling your local fitness center, looking in the phone book under "Personal Training," or asking friends for referrals. Look for a trainer who is certified by the National Strength and Conditioning Association (the top certification for personal trainers) or the American College of Sports Medicine (most often found working in hospital-based fitness centers).

Your Journey Toward Fitness

As a last word, remember that fitness is not something you achieve; it's something you will always work toward. Fitness is not something we eventually "get" and then stop working at: "Use it or you lose it" will always ring true. That's because once you have the sculpted body you want, you must work to maintain it. The good news is that it won't take nearly as much effort to maintain your sculpted look as it did to achieve it. But fitness should still remain a priority in order to live a life filled with strength and vigor. So get to work and stay fit!

The Least You Need to Know

◆ It's better to measure your body-sculpting progress by analyzing body fat percentage than by referring to the scale.

◆ Your local fitness center should offer one or more methods to analyze and track your body fat percentage.

◆ As you get stronger, you'll be able to add more weight to your resistance exercises. This is another way to measure your progress.

◆ Even if you take a temporary hiatus from your body-sculpting routine, you can always jump back in.

◆ A personal trainer can help you set your goals, analyze your progress, or take your program to new levels.

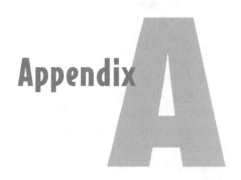

Glossary

aerobic exercise   Activity that raises your heart rate and burns calories. Also known as cardiovascular exercise.

anabolic-androgenic steroids   Man-made substances related to male sex hormones. These drugs are available legally only by prescription to treat conditions that occur when the body produces abnormally low amounts of testosterone, such as delayed puberty and some types of impotence. They are also used to treat loss of lean muscle mass in patients with AIDS and other diseases. *Anabolic* refers to muscle building, and *androgenic* refers to increased masculine characteristics. *Steroids* refers to the class of drugs.

bioelectrical impedence instruments   Tools that measure your body fat via electricity.

body business plan   A clear plan with an ongoing, effective set of short-term steps to help you reach your long-term body-sculpting goals.

body composition   The percentage of fat versus the percentage of lean muscle in your body. Instead of focusing on your weight, measure your body-sculpting goals by analyzing your body composition.

body fat   The cells your body forms to store energy when the calories you eat exceed what your body needs to function. It's otherwise known as flab, cellulite, love handles, and saddlebags.

body sculpting   A philosophy of exercise that incorporates resistance training as part of a complete program to define and tone muscle and shape your body according to your particular goals. For women, this often means losing inches from "problem" areas; for men, if often means gaining inches in areas such as the arms or legs.

calorie   A unit of energy that has been adopted as a simple way for us to compare foods. Zero calories means zero energy, so any calorie-free food or drink is also energy free.

carbohydrate   The primary nutrient/fuel source used by the body during high-intensity activity such as weight training. Carbohydrates (carbs) are used almost exclusively by the brain and nervous systems for energy. Primary sources of carbohydrates are starches and sugars.

combination exercises   Exercises that work different groups of muscles at the same time.

complex carbohydrates   Nutrients that should make up the majority of your carbohydrate intake. Examples are grains, cereals, and vegetables.

crunch   The mainstay of all abdominal exercises. The crunch involves all the muscles in your core.

dietary fat   The amount of fat grams in the food you eat.

driving want   The underlying emotional motivation for achieving your body-sculpting goals.

flexibility   The comfortable range of motion that your joints can move within.

food pyramid   The USDA's recommendations for eating a healthful diet.

heart-rate training zone   Your target heart rate for maximizing your workout. For moderate aerobic exercise, you should aim to elevate your heart rate to 60–80 percent of what it is capable of.

measurable goals   Goals that will enable you to determine on a weekly or monthly basis whether you are making progress or whether you need to adjust your exercise and nutrition routines.

momentum   Movement that's made easier because of uncontrolled speed. Avoid using momentum when doing resistance training.

progression   Consistently intensifying your workout so it remains a challenge to bring continual improvements.

proteins   Nutrients that are the building blocks of the body. They are essential for muscle growth and for keeping all the body's systems working properly.

rating of perceived exertion (RPE)   A means of figuring out the appropriate intensity of your aerobic workout. Shoot for a rating of between 5–6—moderate to somewhat hard—during your workout.

refined sugars   Carbohydrates the body tends to store as fat. These are found in foods such as sodas, candy, and ice cream.

repetition   Reflects each time you complete a full resistance training movement. For example, one ab crunch repetition consists of you crunching up and then lowering your body back to its starting position.

resistance training   Weight-bearing exercises that directly build and strengthen your muscles, bringing you the body-sculpting results you seek.

set   A full sequence of repetitions during resistance training. Doing one to three sets per exercise is the standard recommendation for body sculpting.

set point   The weight your body is comfortable maintaining. Yo-yo dieting has been associated with increasing the body's set point, making it more difficult to reach weight-loss goals.

simple sugars   Carbohydrates that are found naturally in milk products and fruit.

spot reduction   The claim of much (false) advertising that you can reduce body fat in a specific area of the body with exercise. Spot reduction is a myth; the only way to burn fat is through cardiovascular exercise.

spotter A person who watches you do an exercise and takes control of the weight if you suddenly can't.

stability ball A piece of exercise equipment that looks like a highly durable beach ball. It allows you to increase your range of motion on certain exercises.

supplement A food or drink that can help you get enough of the proper nutrients during times when you cannot get them from food alone.

synergy Two or more effective components that, when combined, produce an effect that is greater than each of them alone. For instance, nutrition + flexibility + aerobic exercise + resistance training = better body sculpting results.

tubing Exercise equipment characterized by its long, tubular shape and flexible, rubber band–like qualities.

warm-up Preparing the muscles with some light movement so they're stretched and ready for more intense exercise.

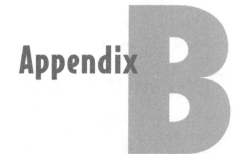

Resources

Home Exercise Equipment

Quest Fitness Solutions
PO Box 546
Nowata, OK 74048
www.quest-fitness-solutions.com

Fitness First
PO Box 251
Shawnee Mission, KS 66201
1-800-421-1791
www.fitness1st.com

M-F Athletic/Perform Better
11 Amflex Dr.
Cranston, RI 02920
1-800-682-6950
www.performbetter.com

Power Systems
2527 Westcott Blvd.
Knoxville, TN 37931
1-800-321-6975
www.power-systems.com

SportsSmith
5925 S. 118th E. Ave.
Tulsa, OK 74146
1-800-713-2880
www.sportsmith.net

Heart-Rate Monitors

Quest Fitness Solutions
PO Box 546
Nowata, OK 74048
www.quest-fitness-solutions.com

Polar Electro
370 Crossways Park Dr.
Woodbury, NY 11797
1-800-290-6330
www.polarusa.com

CardioTech
255 N. Washington St., #202
Rockville, MD 20850
1-800-543-2850
www.cardiotech.net

Nutrition Information

U.S. Department of Agriculture—
Consumer Corner
Official Site of Food, Nutrition, and
Consumer Services
www.nal.usda.gov/fnic/consumersite/
allaboutfood.htm

U.S. Food and Drug Administration (FDA)
5600 Fishers Ln.
Rockville, MD 20857
1-888-463-6332
www.fda.gov

American Dietetic Association
120 S. Riverside Plaza, Suite 2000
Chicago, IL 60606-6995
1-800-877-1600
www.eatright.org

FOOD—Safety, Nutrition, and Preparation
(Sponsored by the University of Nebraska;
includes cooking tips, a free nutrition news-
letter, and other nutrition information.)
lancaster.unl.edu/food

Nutrition Analysis and Tools
(Sponsored by the University of Illinois;
includes a nutrition-analysis tool, an energy
calculator, and links to other nutrition sites.)
nat.crgq.com

Fitness Organizations

American College of Sports Medicine
PO Box 1440
Indianapolis, IN 46206
1-800-486-5643
www.acsm.org

National Strength and Conditioning
Association
PO Box 9908
Colorado Springs, CO 80932
1-800-815-6826
www.nsca-lift.org

President's Council on Physical Fitness
and Sports
200 Independence Ave. S.W., Room 738H
Washington, DC 20201
202-690-9000
www.fitness.gov

International Health, Racquet and Sportsclub
Association (IHRSA)
263 Summer St.
Boston, MA 02210
1-800-228-4772
www.ihrsa.org

Gatorade Sports Science Institute
617 W. Main St.
Barrington, IL 60010
1-800-616-4774
www.gssiweb.com

Nutritional Information

Vitamins: Recommended Daily Allowances (RDA) and Upper Limits (UL) for Adults Over 19 Years Old

Vitamin	RDA	UL	Sources
Biotin	30 ug	ND*	Liver, small amounts in fruits and meats
Choline	550 mg men 425 mg women	3,500 mg	Milk, liver, eggs, peanuts
Folate (Folic acid)	400 ug	1,000 ug	Enriched cereal grains; dark, leafy vegetables; enriched and whole-grain breads and bread products; fortified ready-to-eat cereals
Niacin	16 mg men 14 mg women	35 mg	Meat, fish, poultry, enriched and whole-grain breads and bread products, fortified ready-to-eat cereals
Pantothenic acid	5 mg	ND*	Chicken, beef, potatoes, oats, cereals, tomato products, liver, kidney, yeast, egg yolk, broccoli, whole grains
Riboflavin (vitamin B_2)	1.3 mg men 1.1 mg women	ND*	Organ meats, milk, bread products and fortified cereals
Thiamin (vitamin B_1)	1.2 mg men 1.1 mg women	ND*	Enriched, fortified, or whole-grain products; bread and bread products, mixed foods whose main ingredient is grain; ready-to-eat cereals

Vitamins: Recommended Daily Allowances (RDA) and Upper Limits (UL) for Adults Over 19 Years Old   (continued)

Vitamin	RDA	UL	Sources
Vitamin A	900 ug men 700 ug women	3,000 ug	Liver, dairy products, fish, darkly colored fruits and leafy vegetables
Vitamin B$_6$	1.3 mg men 19–50 yrs 1.7 mg men > 50 yrs 1.3 mg women 19–50 yrs 1.5 mg women > 50 yrs	100 mg	Fortified cereals, organ meats, fortified soy-based meat substitutes
Vitamin B$_{12}$	2.4 ug	ND*	Fortified cereals, meat, fish, poultry
Vitamin C (Ascorbic acid)	90 mg men 75 mg women	2,000 mg	Citrus fruits, tomatoes, tomato juice, potatoes, Brussels sprouts, cauliflower, broccoli, strawberries, cabbage, spinach
Vitamin D (calciferol)	5 ug 19–50 yrs 10 ug 50–70 yrs 15 ug 70 yrs and older	50 ug	Fish liver oils, flesh of fatty fish, liver and fat from seals and polar bears, eggs from hens that have been fed vitamin D, fortified milk products, fortified cereals
Vitamin E	15 mg	1,000 mg	Vegetable oils, unprocessed cereal grains, nuts, fruits, vegetables, meats
Vitamin K	120 ug men 90 ug women	ND*	Green vegetables (collards, spinach, salad greens, broccoli), Brussels sprouts, cabbage, plant oils, margarine

ND—Not determined due to lack of data on adverse effects. Sources should come from foods (no supplements).

Minerals: Recommended Daily Allowances (RDA) and Upper Limits (UL) for Adults Over 19 Years Old

Mineral	RDA	UL	Sources
Calcium	1,000 mg 19–50 yrs 1,200 mg > 50 yrs	2500 mg	Milk, cheese, yogurt, corn tortillas, calcium-set tofu, Chinese cabbage, kale, broccoli
Chromium	35 ug men 19–50 yrs 30 ug men > 50 yrs 25 ug women 19–50 yrs 20 ug women >50 yrs	ND*	Some cereals, meats, poultry, fish, beer
Copper	900 ug	10,000 ug	Organ meats, seafood, nuts, seeds, wheat-bran cereals, whole-grain products, cocoa products

Mineral	RDA	UL	Sources
Iron	8 mg men 18 mg women 19–50 yrs 8 mg women > 50 yrs (post-menopause)	45 mg	Fruits, vegetables, fortified bread and grain products such as cereal, meat, poultry
Magnesium	400 mg men 19–30 yrs 420 mg men > 30 yrs 310 mg women 19–30 yrs 320 mg women > 30 yrs	350 mg (from supplements —no upper limit from food sources)	Green, leafy vegetables; unpolished grains; nuts; meat; starches; milk
Manganese	2.3 mg men 1.8 mg women	11 mg	Nuts, legumes, tea, whole grains
Phosphorus	700 mg	4,000 mg	Milk, yogurt, ice cream, cheese, peas, meat, eggs, some cereals and breads
Selenium	55 ug	400 ug	Organ meats, seafood, plants
Zinc	11 mg men 8 mg women	40 mg	Fortified cereals, red meats, certain seafood

ND—Not determined, due to lack of data on adverse effects. Sources should come from foods (no supplements).

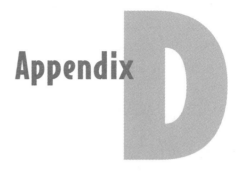

Goals and Logs

You can use the following goal and log sheets exactly as they are, or you can modify them to meet your particular needs. However you decide to journal your goals, exercise, and nutrition, keep accurate records that you can always look back on for help and inspiration.

Long- and Short-Term Goals

Long-term goal (6 months to 1 year from now):

_____

_____

_____

_____

Short-term goals (small pieces of the long-term goal):

Goal #1:

_____

_____

Target date (when you will reach this goal): _____

Daily plan (how you will reach this goal): _____

_____

_____

Goal #2:

_____

_____

Target date: _____

Daily plan: _____

_____

_____

Goal #3:

_____

_____

Target date: _____

Daily plan: _____

_____

_____

Exercise Log

Date:

Aerobic Training:		
Type of Exercise	**Distance/Time/Level**	**Target Heart Rate**
		Heart Rate Maintained:

Resistance Training:			
Exercise:		Exercise:	
Set 1: Reps:	Wt:	Set 1: Reps:	Wt:
Set 2: Reps:	Wt:	Set 2: Reps:	Wt:
Set 3: Reps:	Wt:	Set 3: Reps:	Wt:
Exercise:		Exercise:	
Set 1: Reps:	Wt:	Set 1: Reps:	Wt:
Set 2: Reps:	Wt:	Set 2: Reps:	Wt:
Set 3: Reps:	Wt:	Set 3: Reps:	Wt:
Exercise:		Exercise:	
Set 1: Reps:	Wt:	Set 1: Reps:	Wt:
Set 2: Reps:	Wt:	Set 2: Reps:	Wt:
Set 3: Reps:	Wt:	Set 3: Reps:	Wt:

Daily Nutrition Log

Date:

Food/Drink	Amount/# of Servings	Time	Calories and % Fat

_____

_____

_____

_____

_____

_____

_____

_____

_____

_____

_____

_____

_____

_____

_____

_____

_____

_____

_____

_____

_____

_____

Number of Servings from Each Food Group

Bread, cereal, rice, pasta (6–11): ❑ ❑ ❑ ❑ ❑ ❑ ❑ ❑ ❑ ❑ ❑

Veggies (3–5): ❑ ❑ ❑ ❑ ❑

Fruit (2–4): ❑ ❑ ❑ ❑

Dairy (2–3): ❑ ❑ ❑

Meat, poultry, fish, dry beans, eggs, nuts (2–3): ❑ ❑ ❑

Fats, oils, sweets (as few as possible): ❑ ❑ ❑ ❑ ❑

Glasses of water today (8 oz.): ❑ ❑ ❑ ❑ ❑ ❑ ❑ ❑ ❑ ❑

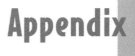

Appendix **E**

Workout Plans

The following workout plans are merely examples of how you can put together your own body-sculpting program. There are literally hundreds of ways of combining workout days, times, and exercises to arrive at the same sculpted look. Your workout should fit your schedule and goals, and most of all, be enjoyable.

Calories Burned with Various Exercises

The numbers that follow are close estimates. The exact number of calories you burn for any activity depends on your weight, your body composition (percent of body fat), and at what intensity level you exercise. To determine how many calories you have burned, multiply your body weight by the calorie figure next to each activity and then multiply by the number of minutes you performed that activity. Add up your activities throughout the day to get a good approximation of how many calories you have burned.

For example:

I rode my bicycle for 30 minutes at 15 mph. I weigh 185 pounds.

185 pounds × .08 × 30 minutes = 444 calories

Activity	Calorie Figure
Aerobics: low-impact	0.044
Aerobics: high-impact	0.056
Aerobics: step, low-impact	0.056
Aerobics: step, high-impact	0.08

Activity	Calorie Figure
Aerobics: water	0.032
Basketball	0.064
Bicycling: 12–13.9 mph	0.064
Bicycling: 14–15.9 mph	0.08
Bicycling: 16–19 mph	0.096
Bicycling: > 19 mph	0.132
Bicycling: BMX/mountain	0.068
Bicycling: stationary: moderate	0.056
Bicycling: stationary: vigorous	0.084
Bowling	0.024
Boxing: sparring	0.072
Calisthenics: moderate	0.036
Calisthenics: vigorous	0.064
Chopping and splitting wood	0.048
Circuit training	0.064
Dancing: disco, ballroom, square	0.044
Dancing: fast, ballet, twist	0.048
Dancing: slow, waltz, fox-trot	0.024
Elliptical trainer	0.072
Flag football	0.064
Gardening	0.036
Golf: carrying clubs	0.044
Golf: using cart	0.028
Handball	0.096
Hiking cross-country	0.048
Hockey: field and ice	0.064
Ice skating	0.056
Inline skating	0.056
Kayaking	0.04
Martial arts	0.08
Moving: carrying boxes	0.056
Mowing lawn: power push mower	0.036
Racquetball: casual	0.056
Racquetball: competitive	0.08
Raking leaves	0.032
Rope jumping	0.08

Activity	Calorie Figure
Rowing: stationary, moderate	0.056
Rowing: stationary, vigorous	0.068
Running: 6 minutes per mile	0.132
Running: 7 minutes per mile	0.116
Running: 8 minutes per mile	0.1
Running: 9 minutes per mile	0.088
Running: 10 minutes per mile	0.08
Running: 12 minutes per mile	0.064
Scuba or skin diving	0.056
Shoveling snow	0.048
Ski machine	0.076
Skiing: cross-country	0.064
Skiing: downhill	0.048
Sleeping	0.005
Sitting: reading or watching TV	0.009
Soccer	0.056
Softball	0.04
Snow shoeing	0.064
Stair step machine	0.048
Stretching, hatha yoga	0.032
Swimming: backstroke	0.064
Swimming: breaststroke	0.08
Swimming: butterfly	0.088
Swimming: crawl (freestyle)	0.088
Tai chi	0.032
Tennis	0.056
Volleyball	0.032
Volleyball: beach	0.064
Volleyball: water	0.024
Walking: 13 minutes per mile	0.04
Walking: 15 minutes per mile	0.036
Walking: 17 minutes per mile	0.032
Water polo	0.08
Water-skiing	0.048
Weight lifting	0.024
Whitewater rafting or kayaking	0.04

Sample Workout Plans

The following workout plans are divided into the number of days a week you want to work out (from two days to six days). The exercise plans describe which body parts you should include each day; it's up to you to decide which exercises you want to use.

Two Days a Week

Plan your workouts on one of these schedules so your workouts are as evenly spaced throughout the week as possible:

- Monday and Thursday
- Tuesday and Friday
- Wednesday and Saturday
- Thursday and Sunday
- Friday and Monday
- Saturday and Tuesday
- Sunday and Wednesday

Include at least one exercise for each muscle group in every workout.

Three Days a Week

Plan your workouts on one of these schedules so your workouts are as evenly spaced throughout the week as possible:

- Monday, Wednesday, and Friday
- Tuesday, Thursday, and Saturday
- Wednesday, Friday, and Sunday
- Thursday, Saturday, and Monday
- Friday, Sunday, and Tuesday
- Saturday, Monday, and Wednesday
- Sunday, Tuesday, and Thursday

Each workout combines muscle groups so you alternate between workout 1 and workout 2. Do not do the same workout twice in a row. Each workout should include at least two exercises for each muscle group.

- **Workout 1:** chest, triceps, shoulders, abs
- **Workout 2:** thighs, biceps, glutes, calves, back

Four Days a Week

You now have two workout days in a row; to ensure adequate rest, plan your workouts on one of these schedules:

- Monday, Tuesday, Thursday, and Friday
- Tuesday, Wednesday, Friday, and Saturday
- Wednesday, Thursday, Saturday, and Sunday
- Thursday, Friday, Sunday, and Monday
- Friday, Saturday, Monday, and Tuesday
- Saturday, Sunday, Tuesday, and Wednesday
- Sunday, Monday, Wednesday, and Thursday

Each workout combines muscle groups so you alternate between workout 1 and workout 2. Do not do the same workout twice in a row. Each workout should include at least two exercises for each muscle group.

- **Workout 1:** chest, triceps, shoulders, abs
- **Workout 2:** thighs, biceps, glutes, calves, back

Five Days a Week

You have three workouts in a row, a day of rest, two workouts in a row, and a day of rest—then repeat. Plan your workouts on one of these schedules:

- Monday, Tuesday, Wednesday, Friday, and Saturday

◆ Tuesday, Wednesday, Thursday, Saturday, and Sunday

◆ Wednesday, Thursday, Friday, Sunday, and Monday

◆ Thursday, Friday, Saturday, Monday, and Tuesday

◆ Friday, Saturday, Sunday, Tuesday, and Wednesday

◆ Saturday, Sunday, Monday, Wednesday, and Thursday

◆ Sunday, Monday, Tuesday, Thursday, and Friday

Each workout combines muscle groups so you complete workouts 1, 2, and 3 on consecutive days; then start back at workout 1. Do not do the same workout twice in a row. Each workout should include at least three exercises for each muscle group.

◆ **Workout 1:** chest, triceps, shoulders
◆ **Workout 2:** thighs, glutes, calves
◆ **Workout 3:** biceps, back, shoulders

Six Days a Week

Plan your schedule so you have one day off after every three workouts. For example, exercise on Monday, Tuesday, and Wednesday; take Thursday off; work out on Friday, Saturday, and Sunday; and take Monday off. Keep repeating three days "on" and one day "off."

Each workout combines muscle groups so you complete workouts 1, 2, and 3 on consecutive days, and then start back at workout 1. Do not do the same workout twice in a row. Each workout should include at least three exercises for each muscle group.

◆ **Workout 1:** chest, triceps, shoulders
◆ **Workout 2:** thighs, glutes, calves
◆ **Workout 3:** biceps, back, shoulders

Sample Workout Progressions

As a general rule, move from easier to more complex exercises as you master each movement. Here are some examples by muscle group:

◆ **Abs:** basic crunch, double crunch, stability ball crunch

◆ **Chest:** modified push-up, push-up, dumbbell press, bench press

◆ **Back:** tubing row, seated row machine, barbell row

◆ **Shoulders:** machine shoulder press, tubing press, dumbbell press

◆ **Biceps:** dumbbell curl, concentration curl, seated ball tubing curl

◆ **Triceps:** dumbbell kickback, overhead press, dumbbell French curl

◆ **Glutes:** horizontal leg lifts, squat and lift, tubing lateral lift

◆ **Thighs:** body squat, leg press machine, barbell squat

◆ **Calves:** seated calf raise, standing calf raise, calf raise machine

Index

X–Y–Z

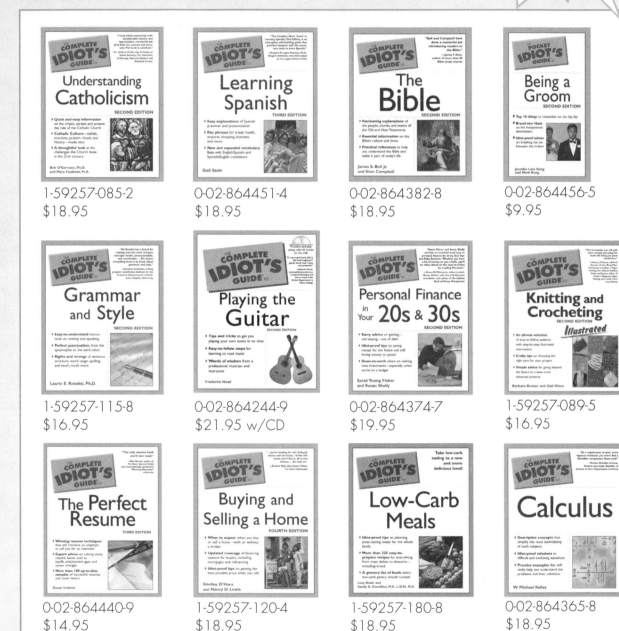